# OPTIMIZING HEALTH
### and
# CANCER OUTCOMES
### with
# FUNCTIONAL MEDICINE

## BRIAN LAWENDA, M.D.

ISBNs:
Kindle: 979-8-9883448-1-0
Print: 979-8-9883448-0-3

Editor: Siobhan Gallagher
Cover artist: Tamian Wood, Beyond Design International
Type setting: Codruț Sebastian Făgăraș

*This book is dedicated to all of the brave, resilient cancer patients and survivors who have inspired me to delve deeper into the world of integrative oncology and functional medicine. Your strength and determination to take control of your health and well-being has been a constant source of motivation for me.*

*I also want to express my gratitude to the numerous experts in these fields who have shared their knowledge and insights with me. Through their guidance and teachings, I have learned how functional medicine testing and addressing abnormal results may impact health outcomes in our oncology patients and cancer survivors. From addressing nutrient deficiencies to gut microbiome dysbiosis, I have seen firsthand how these interventions can improve overall health and well-being in individuals with cancer or a history of cancer.*

*I hope that this book serves as a helpful resource for both healthcare professionals who care for those with cancer and for cancer patients and survivors looking to take a more holistic and personalized data-oriented approach to their care. Thank you for allowing me to be a part of your journey toward optimal health and wellness.*

# Table of Contents

# Introduction

*Optimizing Health and Cancer Outcomes with Functional Medicine* is the companion guide to another book, one I co-authored with nutritionist Conner Middelmann that takes an overarching, holistic approach to dealing with cancer: *Empowered Against Cancer*. (See the Resources section at the end of the book.)

*Empowered Against Cancer* contains both medical and dietary advice as a more overarching treatment approach, where patients take an active role in their own treatment, while this book focuses more closely on testing and treatment options.

## Patients who are more actively engaged in their treatment and in optimizing their health report more positive outcomes

With that in mind, *Empowered Against Cancer* covers the basic tenets of integrative oncology approaches to cancer care.

I recommend, in addition to reading *Empowered Against Cancer*, that you read this guide as early in your journey as you can, so you can familiarize yourself with various testing and treatment options available to you. (By all means share a copy of this companion guide with your doctor or care providers.) You needn't dwell too much the first time around on the more technical information—you can go back and review the details later. Instead, I recommend that you first read it to get a sense of the path you might want to take in your particular situation, as everyone's situation—and cancer—is different. Discuss the various tests with your physician so you can chart a plan together.

In this companion guidebook, I explain how to use functional medicine testing (which examines one's nutritional status, systemic inflammation, metabolic health, chronic stress, and much more) and other state-of-the-art testing to assess the particular risk factors you may have that can potentially contribute to cancer development, progression, and possible recurrence. I also share valuable information with you on various state-of-the-art tests that have been shown to be useful in identifying whether you have a genetic risk for developing numerous cancers as well as enhancing your healthcare provider's ability to detect the presence or progression of an existing cancer sooner than standard traditional tests and exams can.

Moving from diagnosis to treatment, this book also discusses functional tumor sensitivity testing, which helps to identify which drugs have the greatest chance of being effective against your cancer.

Even if you are fortunate enough to be in remission, it is important to know that many patients in remission are still confronted by an increased risk of cardiovascular disease. With that in mind, I have also included for you a section on how to assess your cardiovascular disease risks, as this is important for every cancer survivor to know.

Let's get started.

# Cancer Care Guidelines from the Experts

The National Comprehensive Cancer Network, *www.nccn. org*, has published a set of general guidelines, which are evidence-based recommendations developed by experts to help oncologists determine the best treatment options for their cancer patients. Among the many consensus-based guidelines, the NCCN is the most widely used guideline and has recommendations for the majority of cancer types.

While their professional guidelines can be accessed by any healthcare provider, the NCCN also has another set of guidelines, written specifically for patients, that you can access for free. There, they offer information about the various types of cancers, as well as other factors to consider when planning a treatment approach.

Before your oncologist meets with you for the first time, or when you return to them for follow-up appointments, rest assured that they are familiar with the NCCN's guidelines pertaining to your diagnosis. These guidelines are consistently updated, so each time any of your cancer care team providers consult the guidelines, they access the latest information available.

The guidelines cover such topics as the recommended workup, how to stage your particular cancer type, treatment recommendations, how to manage any recurrence or metastatic disease, and how to best track it and follow up.

These guidelines are a good overall guidance, but think of them, perhaps, as more as a set of directions versus a comprehensive roadmap or GPS which endeavors to give you a more complete picture of the routes you can take. This book, and its predecessor, *Empowered Against Cancer*, include a lot of information that does not appear in the NCCN guidelines. Instead, the guidelines and these books complement and support one another.

# Second Opinions

As a patient, you always have the right to seek a second opinion on your care, whether you do it right at the start or at any time during your treatment. You should never feel guilty about this, and no one should ever make you feel guilty about wanting to do this.

No doubt your physician has had patients come to them seeking a second opinion (or even a third), as well as having had their patients obtain one elsewhere. You need to feel confident that you have been diagnosed correctly and be made aware of all of your treatment options before you proceed. You want to be assured that your doctor is doing everything possible for you.

If your doctor becomes upset over your obtaining a second opinion, or even expressing the desire to get one, they are not the right healthcare provider for you. It is the job of your physician to help you achieve the best outcome possible, regardless of where and by whom you obtain that care. In fact, a study of data collected as far back as 1992 revealed that 56% of cancer patients had obtained second opinions.[1]

If you have been diagnosed with cancer, it is important that you feel comfortable with the specialists on your cancer care team and what they recommend. In most cases, you can take the time to do your research and get additional opinions without negatively impacting the effectiveness of your

---

[1] Hewitt, Breen & Devesa, "Cancer prevalence and survivorship issues: analyses of the 1992 National Health Interview Survey," pubmed.ncbi.nlm.nih.gov/10469749.

treatment. It's important to recognize that even if you have already started treatment, it's never too late to get a second opinion. In fact, you are entitled to obtain second opinions at any time after diagnosis or during your care.

Many patients seek second opinions to make sure they have the most accurate diagnosis. In a study[2] of breast cancer patients, more than half of them changed their treatment after getting a second opinion from a group of medical specialists. If you feel that your diagnosis is unclear, or that your team can't make a diagnosis, you should get a second opinion. A study[3] from the Mayo Clinic found that patients who got second opinions under these conditions ended up receiving a new or refined diagnosis *88% of the time.*

Examples of when you might get a second opinion:
- Pathology second opinions: These can be important because they can change your treatment plan. For example, one study[4] found that 11% of breast cancer pathology second opinions resulted in significant differences.

- Radiology second opinions: Your oncology team relies heavily on the radiology interpretation of your studies. This is because the radiology findings can lead to recommendations for further diagnostic tests or treatment plans, such as biopsies, surgeries, radiation therapy, and systemic therapies.

- Radiation Oncology, Medical Oncology and Surgical second opinions: Times when it is a good idea to get a second opinion include cases where you might need radiation oncology, medical oncology, or surgical treatment. It is common for specialists to have different opinions on how to treat someone. For example, surgeons might have different opinions on the best way to approach a surgery, medical oncologists might

---

2   www.breastcancer.org/research-news/20061130b.

3   onlinelibrary.wiley.com/doi/10.1111/jep.12747/full.

4   pubmed.ncbi.nlm.nih.gov/25273328.

choose different drug regimens, and some might discuss clinical trial options more often.

- Academic expert second opinions: If you have a rare cancer type and none of the members of your cancer care team are experts in your specific cancer, it is a good idea to at least consider getting evaluated at a center of excellence that specializes in your condition. Studies show that higher-volume specialty centers may have better outcomes, especially with less common conditions.

- If any of your cancer team providers seem unsure about the type or stage of your cancer.

- If your oncology team offers you more than one option to treat your cancer and you're not sure which choice is best.

- If you are having difficulty communicating with any of your physicians, if you feel rushed in your encounters, or just do not feel comfortable with them.

- If the treatment you are receiving is no longer working and your doctor tells you they can't do anything else.

- If your treatment seems too toxic, or you experience serious side effects, and your doctors do not change your treatment.

- If you hear about other treatment options for your condition, and your physician either doesn't know about them or doesn't address whether they might be helpful.

- If your interest lies in an integrative oncology approach to your cancer care, and this is not available with the group of providers you are currently seeing, you should consult with a center or integrative oncology provider that offers this service, such as myself. I offer both in-office and remote options (*ioeprogram.com/consultations*).

- Are you choosing a naturopathic physician (N.D.) to be part of your health care team? Ask the N.D. if they have expertise in working with cancer patients. You can find a list of oncology-specialized N.D.s through the Oncology Association of Naturopathic Physicians website, *oncanp.org*.
- If your cancer is not responding to your oncologist's recommended drugs, consider getting a chemosensitivity test conducted on your cancer to find out which cancer drugs will likely be the most effective in the treatment of your cancer (see the chapter on Chemosensitivity Assays, page 83).

Make sure to involve your cancer care team when getting a second opinion, as the second opinion team will need access to all of your medical records. This is so they can give you the best advice possible. Some of the records that are typically requested include radiology studies and reports, pathology specimens and reports, laboratory reports, and consultation and office encounter notes from your cancer care team providers.

Obtain copies of all of your medical records *before* you go to get a second opinion. This will help avoid delays. I also recommend making additional copies of these records for your personal files. Medical facilities usually send records ahead of time after a request has been made, but it is best to carry copies with you, just in case the originals are lost during transit.

There are many resources you can use to figure out where to go for a second opinion:

- Start by asking the members of your cancer care team where they would go, and which specialist they would recommend you see.
- You may know people personally who have been diagnosed and treated for a similar cancer who can tell you about the providers they recommend.

- You can also search online for experts who are faculty of a National Cancer Institute (NCI) designated cancer center (*www.cancer.gov/research/nci-role/cancer-centers*). These experts are on staff of programs recognized by the NCI as the top academic cancer centers in the U.S. You can also call the NCI Cancer Information Service (1-800-4-CANCER) or consult online with an information specialist through its LiveHelp feature, *livehelp.cancer.gov*.
- Cancer support groups and online cancer discussion boards can help direct you to recommended specialists.
- Integrative oncology consults can also be done, e.g.:
  - *IOEProgram.com* (Dr. Lawenda's consultation service and program)
  - *themossreport.com*
  - Other providers (see *glennsabin.com/integrative-oncology-providers*)

Many insurance providers, including Medicare, will pay for a second opinion from a doctor who is not in your insurance network. If you are unable to afford to travel for a second opinion, there may be patient assistance programs that can help.

If the second opinion is the same as the first opinion, you will feel surer about what to do. You will have to decide which center or provider you want to use for treatment. If there are differences in the two opinions, you have a few options on what to do next:

- Discuss the second opinion with your first-opinion providers, and ask them their thoughts on it. I find that is often very helpful to ask them to communicate directly with each other to see if they can come to an agreement.
- Obtain a third opinion from another specialist, and ask them to review the first two opinions and give you their recommendation. As always, it is best if the consulted

specialists can call each other to discuss your case. You have a right to ask them to do so.

- Conduct your own research by referring to the following expert panel recommended guidelines:
  - National Comprehensive Cancer Network (NCCN), *www.nccn.org/patientresources/patient-resources/guidelines-for-patients*
  - National Cancer Institute PDQ (Physician Data Query), *www.cancer.gov/publications/pdq*

In the end, you will need to base your decision on the different recommendations, programs, and providers you consult. If the opinions significantly differ—and that can happen—then it is likely that, in your particular situation, there is no one right answer. You must make the best choice for you based on your circumstances and the information you have.

Do not feel obligated to seek a second opinion if you trust your doctors and agree with their diagnosis and treatment plan. And, remember, you can always request a second opinion at a later date.

# Functional Medicine

Functional medicine is a science-based approach to disease management that centers on health and wellness, is based primarily on lifestyle modifications and non-pharmaceutical interventions, and is guided by lab testing and pertinent clinical research findings. Rather than focusing on treating your *symptoms*, functional medicine attempts to identify and treat many of the *root causes* of chronic health problems.

Functional medicine is a tool that I use to assess a patient's biological state, as this influences how your cancer develops, its growth, metastatic spread, and risk of recurrence. It's important to know that it is uncommon for oncologists to receive functional medicine training as part of their education in conventional medicine, which is why many of my patients have not already been tested for these potential issues before coming to see me.

This figure shows you how multiple variables can potentially promote the development, progression, or recurrence of cancer. We have the ability to assess each of these variables through functional medicine lab testing and track them over time.

**Functional Medicine Testing to Identify Factors That May Indirectly Influence Cancer Development, Growth, Metastasis and Recurrence**

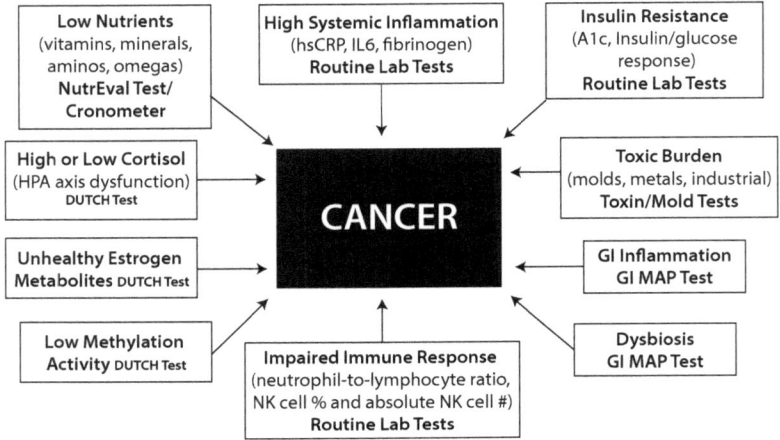

| | | |
|---|---|---|
| **Low Nutrients** (vitamins, minerals, aminos, omegas) **NutrEval Test/ Cronometer** | **High Systemic Inflammation** (hsCRP, IL6, fibrinogen) **Routine Lab Tests** | **Insulin Resistance** (A1c, Insulin/glucose response) **Routine Lab Tests** |
| **High or Low Cortisol** (HPA axis dysfunction) DUTCH Test | **CANCER** | **Toxic Burden** (molds, metals, industrial) **Toxin/Mold Tests** |
| **Unhealthy Estrogen Metabolites** DUTCH Test | | **GI Inflammation GI MAP Test** |
| **Low Methylation Activity** DUTCH Test | **Impaired Immune Response** (neutrophil-to-lymphocyte ratio, NK cell % and absolute NK cell #) **Routine Lab Tests** | **Dysbiosis GI MAP Test** |

There are a few helpful tests that I recommend to many of my patients. The test(s) you choose will depend on your symptoms, your past medical history, and what the test itself is designed to show. Below is my list of recommended types of tests for some of the most common areas many people want to explore when they seek testing.

- **Micronutrients** – NutrEval Plasma test (Genova Diagnostics) assesses your body's levels of vitamins, minerals, amino acids, fatty acids, and any toxic metals

- **Insulin resistance** – hbA1c and glucose tolerance test with insulin

- **GI (gastrointestinal) health** – GI MAP test (Diagnostic Solutions Laboratory) or GI Effects Comprehensive Stool Profile (Genova Diagnostics) assesses for gut inflammation, leaky gut, digestive enzymes, blood, dysbiosis (microbial imbalances), and parasites

- **Systemic inflammation** – high sensitivity CRP (hsCRP), fibrinogen and IL-6

- **Hypothalamic-pituitary-adrenal axis** – designed to gauge the interaction between these three important glands inside you, the DUTCH test (dried urine test for comprehensive hormones by Precision Analytical) assesses your levels of cortisol, sex hormone metabolites, methylation, and melatonin

- **Immune status** – NK (natural killer) cell assay (the job of your NK cells is to target and eliminate tumors inside you); and a CBC (complete blood count) with differential, to calculate your neutrophil-to-lymphocyte ratio)

- **Toxin/mold status** – GPL-TOX Profile and MycoTOX Profile (Mosaic Diagnostics, formerly Great Plains Laboratory), which assess your exposure to many toxins and molds.

- **Heavy metals testing** – Mercury Tri-Test & Blood Metals Panel, by Quicksilver Scientific

# Immune Function

The immune system is one of the most complex systems in our bodies. It mainly consists of our white blood cells, antibodies, signaling proteins, lymphatic-rich tissues and vessels, and our microbiome. Depending on the circumstances, these cells, signaling proteins, and microorganisms can either promote or suppress tumor development and progression. For example, if you have an acute bacterial or viral infection, you will typically see your immune system activity upregulated, meaning that you'll see elevated levels of white blood cells and inflammatory proteins. While this systemic immune response is normal—and desirable—when it comes to battling acute infections, you don't want chronic, long-term elevated levels after the infection has resolved. Persistently high immune stimulation can sometimes lead to auto-immune conditions (where your immune system mistakenly attacks specific tissues and organs it shouldn't) or, more commonly, a diminished immune response ("immune exhaustion") against infectious organisms and cancer.

While we can't easily measure all of these immune components, because they are numerous and complex, we can employ some of the more important associated lab tests to gain a basic understanding of our anticancer immune status. The following lab tests provide insights into your general immune status.

**Neutrophil-to-lymphocyte ratio, or NLR** – this ratio has been well established as a predictor of cancer outcomes. In the past decade, researchers have analyzed the association between NLR and cancer outcomes. NLR is the ratio of absolute neutrophils to absolute lymphocytes, two types of white blood cells that are part of the immune system. The NLR is obtained through a complete blood count (CBC) with differential by simply dividing the number of absolute neutrophils by the number of absolute lymphocytes. While an optimal NLR value has not been defined, most studies suggest that a high NLR (range: >2–5) is associated with worse cancer outcomes.

## Anticancer Immune System Activity
### Neutrophil:Lymphocyte Ratio (NLR)

NLR reflects the balance between two aspects of the immune system: acute inflammation (as indicated by the neutrophil count) and adaptive immunity (lymphocyte count).

Higher neutrophils: acute inflammation and infections

Optimal NLR defined variably in different studies, but most indicate that better cancer outcomes are seen with an NLR 2–5

https://bmcresnotes.biomedcentral.com/articles/10.1186/s13104-016-2335-5

**Natural killer (NK) cells** – NK cells are the most abundant immune cell in the body. They identify, attack, and kill diseased cells. They also play a critical role in preventing cancer. When a healthy cell mutates into a cancerous one, NK cells often destroy it. That's why the level of NK cells is one of the most important markers to monitor cancer risk and immune response to viruses and bacteria. Having a normal range of NK cells correlates with improved responses against infections and cancer.

In ideal circumstances, your immune system detects cancer cells, produces antibodies that target them, and deploys cancer-killing cells throughout the body to destroy them. This complex process is happening all the time, which is critical, as all of us have cancer cells constantly developing in our body. The mere fact that not everyone gets diagnosed with cancer in their lifetime is a testament in large part to how well their immune system functions.

It is also well established that having an impaired immune system is a risk factor for developing cancer, and worse cancer outcomes. We see this in individuals with immunodeficiency diseases, those on immune-suppressive drugs, or those with conditions that impair immunity, such as obesity, nutrient deficiencies, chronic systemic inflammation, chronic stress, gut dysbiosis, and insulin resistance.

Numerous physiological variables can impact one's immune function. Functional medicine assay testing can be used to assess many of these. For example:

- Micronutrient assays measure levels of vitamins, minerals, amino acids, and fatty acids and identifies deficiencies that can impair immune function and increase chronic systemic inflammation.

- An oral glucose tolerance test with insulin levels and a hemoglobin A1C (HbA1c or A1c) can identify insulin resistance and diabetes mellitus, which impair the body's ability to respond to infections and are associated with poorer cancer outcomes.

- Elevated inflammatory markers such as C-reactive protein (CRP), fibrinogen, certain interleukins (such as IL-6), and others are associated with impaired immune function and increased risks for infection and cancer.
- Gut DNA microbiome testing measures the diversity and quantity of microorganisms in your intestines. High or low levels (significantly above or below the normal reference ranges) and low diversity of these microorganisms is called "dysbiosis" and can lead to a weaker immune system, nutrient deficiencies, and chronic systemic inflammation.
- Hypothalamic-pituitary-adrenal (HPA) axis testing assesses cortisol levels, a stress hormone that, when either too high or too low (referred to as "HPA axis dysfunction"), can lead to impaired immune function, insulin resistance and chronic systemic inflammation.

## Optimizing Immune Function

It is fundamentally important to assess and address your immune health in terms of your overall cancer and health outcomes. As a clinician, I am frequently asked by patients how they can improve their immune function. To answer this question, it is crucial to start with the basics: What factors affect the immune system?

There are many factors that affect immune function, such as gut health, nutrient status, stress levels, sleep quality and quantity, exercise, and toxic exposures.

## A Functional Medicine Approach to Optimize Anti-Cancer Immune Activity
### Low Anti-Cancer Immune Response

Dark Gray boxes: Undergo tests to provide your neutrophil-to-lymphocyte ratio (NLR) and the number of NK cells in your blood

| Neutrophil-to-Lymphocyte Ratio >2 | Normal NK Cell % and Absolute NK Cell # |
|---|---|

Medium Gray boxes: If NLR is high and NK cell numbers are low:

| Immune Supportive Supplements & Nutrients | Stress Management | Sleep | Exercise |
|---|---|---|---|

Light Gray boxes: Assess and address other variables that can impact immune function through functional medicine testing:

| High Systemic Inflammation | Nutrient Deficiencies | High Toxin & Mold Burden |
|---|---|---|
| HPA Axis Dysfunction | Dysbiosis, Leaky Gut, Gut Inflammation, Food Sensitivities | Insulin Resistance |

Immune system optimization is done by performing a root cause analysis to identify modifiable variables that may be contributing to one's impaired immune activity and then devising a plan, or protocol, to manage these issues. I start by assessing my patient's HPA axis (the DUTCH test), systemic inflammation (hsCRP, fibrinogen, and IL-6), insulin resistance (A1c and a glucose tolerance test with insulin), nutrient status (NutrEval test), gut health status (GI MAP test), and any toxic burden (Mosaic Diagnostics toxin tests).

Any abnormalities identified by these tests need to be addressed using a multipronged approach. Examples of interventions might include minimizing toxic exposures, stress management, sleep optimization, regular exercise, replacing nutrient deficiencies, addressing insulin resistance, and gut health. Taking certain supplements, such as adaptogens (botanical compounds and mushrooms that help normalize high or low cortisol levels resulting from chronic stress) and micronutrients, can also be very helpful.

Don't discount the importance of assessing and addressing your immune health when it comes to your overall cancer and health outcomes.

# Chronic Systemic Inflammation

Inflammation is a normal response by your body that occurs any time there is damage to or abnormality in cells. It can be acute, lasting for days to weeks, such as with a healing wound, bruise, burn or bacterial infection; or the inflammation can be chronic, resulting from conditions which can last for months to years, such as certain viral infections (e.g., HPV (human papilloma virus), hepatitis C, Epstein-Barr), intestinal dysbiosis, nutrient deficiencies, and HPA axis dysfunction.

Your body attempts to repair cellular injury and inflammation through the release of proteins, like cytokines such as interferon and interleukin, which don't just act locally but also have effects on cells throughout your body. This can manifest with many symptoms, such as fatigue, depression, pain, diarrhea, or constipation, for example.

If the inflammatory process does not self-resolve within days to weeks of its onset, chronic inflammation will develop. It is chronic systemic inflammation that has adverse, potentially serious effects on our bodies. Many factors contribute to chronic inflammation, including but not limited to impaired immunity, insufficient physical activity, low muscle mass, obesity, gut dysbiosis (an imbalance of gut microbes), poor diet, chronic stress, disturbed or insufficient sleep, exposure to environmental toxins, and tobacco and/or alcohol use.

Chronic systemic inflammation often involves the activation of a protein called NF Kappa B, which can promote the growth, spread, and recurrence of cancer. NF Kappa B activation can also reduce the effectiveness of many cancer therapies.

The next figure, on page 20, breaks down the many causes of chronic inflammation and shows how they interact. It also illustrates how numerous conditions can occur as a result of when you suffer from chronic inflammation, such as type 2 diabetes, cardiovascular disease, cancer, depression, non-alcoholic fatty liver disease, cardiovascular disease, autoimmune diseases (such as rheumatoid arthritis), neurodegenerative diseases (such as Alzheimer's), sarcopenia (muscle loss), osteoporosis (bone loss), and impaired immunity.

We can measure the degree of chronic systemic inflammation with blood biomarkers such as high-sensitivity C-reactive protein (hsCRP), fibrinogen, and IL-6. Studies have shown that elevated levels of these biomarkers correlate with worse health outcomes, so tracking these over time is a useful way to assess how you are doing in addressing your overall chronic systemic inflammatory state.

## Assessing Inflammation

The most common tests I order to assess the overall chronic inflammatory state in my patients include:
- hsCRP (high-sensitivity C-reactive protein)
- IL-6 (interleukin-6)
- Fibrinogen

## Reversing Chronic Systemic Inflammation

Once we've determined whether or not you have chronic systemic inflammation, we can address this using a multipronged approach.

### A Functional Medicine Approach to Reduce Systemic Inflammation

Systemic Inflammation

Dark Gray boxes: Start by assessing elevated levels of inflammation markers

| hsCRP | Fibrinogen | IL-6 |
|---|---|---|

Medium Gray boxes: Address these potential contributors to systemic inflammation

| Minimize Toxins and Molds | Minimize Body Fat | Anti-Inflammatory Supportive Supplements and Nutrients | |
|---|---|---|---|
| Stress Management | Increase Muscle Mass | Sleep | Exercise |

Light Gray boxes: Consider functional medicine testing for potential contributing factors to systemic inflammation

| Dysbiosis, Leaky Gut, Gut Inflammation, Food Sensitivities | Low Methylation |
|---|---|
| HPA axis dysfunction | Nutrient Deficiencies |
| Insulin Resistance | High Toxin and Mold Burden |

Chronic systemic inflammation is the result of a complex interplay among many factors, including lifestyle, environment, genetics, and any other underlying health conditions.

In order to address chronic systemic inflammation, I first test for the most common causative factors. These include nutrient deficiencies, HPA axis dysfunction, insulin resistance, gut health problems, toxins, methylation status, and overweight/underweight status. Then, after we've identified any problems through testing, we start by addressing them with lifestyle and non-pharmacologic interventions.

Having chronic systemic inflammation is a biological risk factor, not a requirement, for cancer or other chronic diseases, but it is often present in individuals with these conditions. This is why it's so important to assess and address this in all individuals who want to optimize their health and cancer outcomes using a functional medicine approach to their cancer care.

# Insulin Resistance

Testing our patients for insulin resistance is one of the most critical pathophysiological processes that we can assess and manage that can impact cancer and numerous health outcomes. Glucose is the predominant fuel for most cancer cells and insulin is a known cancer growth factor. It has been well established that patients with insulin resistance and type 2 diabetes have a higher incidence of developing many cancers, as well as worse cancer outcomes.

Insulin regulates the glucose in our bodies. Glucose is used by most cells, but the channel that glucose takes to enter them needs to be "unlocked" first. Insulin acts as the key to unlock that channel, permitting glucose to enter.

If you have insulin resistance, those channels don't open as easily, which leads to higher blood glucose levels. This resulting glucose elevation is sensed by the pancreas, which releases more insulin into the circulation to push even harder on those channels in order to drive glucose levels down.

What does that mean for you? Your body stores most of its excess glucose as fat, so an excess of glucose and insulin leads to an increased number of adipocytes—fat cells. These adipocytes can start to accumulate in organs and tissues, causing dysfunction of their normal functions. When your body can no longer produce more adipocytes (a genetically predetermined state called a "personal fat threshold"), your existing fat cells get larger (adipocyte hypertrophy) in an attempt to house all of this excess glucose as fat. As these fat cells get larger, they trigger a low-grade local (in the fat tissue) and systemic inflammatory response, which can negatively affect many physiological processes throughout your body. Furthermore, the increase in visceral fat, the fat that surrounds organs, serves as a source of estrogen production, which can stimulate the growth of estrogen-sensitive cells, something that is a concern for patients who have cancers that have overexpression of estrogen receptors, like estrogen-receptor-positive breast cancers.

These overly large (hypertrophic) fat cells can be found in a number of places: around blood vessels and the heart, which increases your risk for atherosclerosis and cardiovascular disease; inside the liver, which leads to a fatty liver and liver inflammation; and inside the pancreas, which leads to beta cell dysfunction (beta cells are pancreatic cells that produce and release insulin, so when beta cells no longer function properly, insulin production can decline) and insulin-dependent diabetes.

This increase in systemic inflammation can suppress your immune system (through immune exhaustion) and promote gut dysbiosis (imbalance of gut microorganisms), HPA axis dysfunction (HPA is your hypothalamic–pituitary–adrenal system, a stress hormone signaling system), insulin resistance, cancer cell spread (metastases), growth, and more. In a nutshell, when you approach your personal fat threshold, systemic inflammation rises, increasing the risk for numerous serious conditions, such as cancer and cardiovascular disease.

As illustrated in the next figure, many studies have shown that individuals with higher blood sugar and higher insulin levels have faster tumor progression, increased risk of recurrence and metastases, and worse cancer survival and overall survival outcomes. Data indicate that all-cause mortality rates rise rapidly in those who have fasting glucose levels greater than 100 milligrams per deciliter and a hemoglobin A1C value greater than 5–6%.

## Relationship Between Fasting Glucose and Overall Mortality

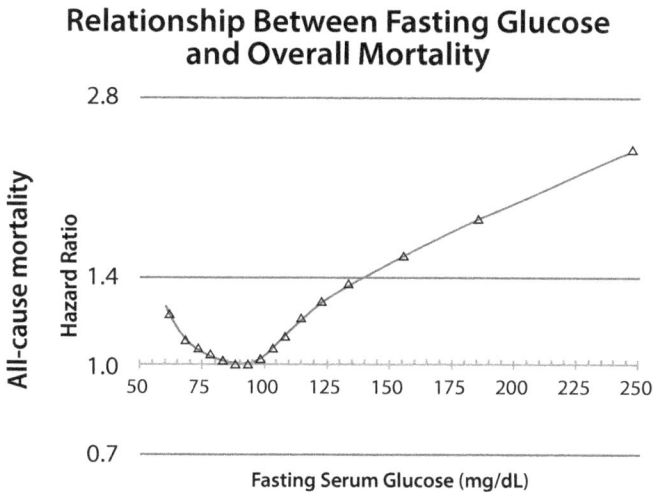

Lowest risk of dying from any cause: a fasting glucose of 76–99 mg/dL

https://pubmed.ncbi.nlm.nih.gov/28811570/

## Assessing Insulin Resistance

The two tests I commonly order to assess for insulin resistance are:

- Hemoglobin A1c (or simply A1c)
- Glucose tolerance test with insulin (or insulin-glucose tolerance test)

Classically, a hemoglobin A1c within the normal range is considered to be below 5.7%, prediabetes range 5.7–6.4% and diabetes range 6.5% or higher. Studies show that as the A1c rises above 5–6%, individuals experience worse health and cancer outcomes.

In addition to the hemoglobin A1C test, the gold standard for assessing insulin resistance is the glucose tolerance test with insulin. This test takes up to two hours and requires you to fast the night before, for eight hours, before drawing your blood to test your insulin and glucose levels. (Consuming food or beverages other than water before the test causes the glucose levels in your blood to rise naturally, and distort the results. This test is also often inaccurate in those on a ketogenic diet). That first blood draw provides a baseline level of what your fasting blood glucose and insulin levels are.

Immediately following the blood draw, you are given a beverage to drink that contains a high level of glucose, after which your insulin and glucose levels are checked again. This is repeated several times over the next two hours to gauge the rate at which your insulin and glucose rises and falls, indicating whether or not you have insulin resistance.

## Ideal Target Ranges

| | |
|---|---|
| A1C | Less than or equal to 5.4% (ideally </=5.1%) |
| Insulin–Glucose Response Test (optimal values) | |
| Fasting glucose | <90 mg/dl |
| Fasting insulin | <6 mIU/dl |
| Glucose 1 hour after glucose drink | <130 mg/dl (ideally, no more than 40 mg/dl above the fasting level) |
| Glucose 2 hours after glucose drink | <100 mg/dl |
| Insulin 1 hour after glucose drink | <30 mIU/dl |
| Insulin 2 hours after glucose drink | <20 mIU/dl |

You can also purchase a finger-stick glucose monitor, or a continuous glucose monitor, to assess your blood sugar response to foods and other stimuli (stress, sleep, exercise, etc.), and track this over time. As with the insulin-glucose response test, if you are tracking your sugars with a glucose meter, you ideally want to fall within these thresholds:
- Fasting glucose:              <90 mg/dl
- Glucose 1 hour after meals:   <130 mg/dl
- Glucose 2 hours after meals:  <100 mg/dl

If your levels are higher than this, I highly recommend tracking and modifying your diet with the guidance of a dietitian or nutritionist, or purchasing what I consider to be a fantastic online course called "Data Driven Fasting" (*www.datadrivenfasting.com*) that teaches you how to use blood sugar testing to reverse insulin resistance.

## A Functional Medicine Approach to Reduce Insulin Resistance

### Insulin Resistance

Dark Gray boxes: Start by undergoing insulin resistance lab tests.

| HBA1C | Insulin-Glucose Response Test | Fingerstick or Continuous Glucose Monitor | |
|---|---|---|---|

Medium Gray boxes: If insulin resistance is an issue:

| Increase Muscle Mass | | Supportive Supplements, Nutrients or Drugs | |
|---|---|---|---|
| Exercise | | Manage Stress | |
| Minimize Body Fat | | Sleep | Cronometer |

Light Gray boxes: Consider functional medicine testing to identify contributing factors to your insulin resistance

| Systemic Inflammation | High Toxin and Mold Burden |
|---|---|
| HPA Axis Dysfunction | Gut Dysbiosis |
| Nutrient Deficiencies | |

Visceral fat loss and building muscle mass are among the most important management tools to address insulin resistance. To lose visceral body fat requires reducing calorie intake, increasing physical activity, reducing stress, and improving sleep quality. When you build muscle mass, you increase your body's glycogen (a small amount of glucose that can be stored in the liver and muscle as glycogen and later converted back into glucose when needed for energy), storage capacity, and basal metabolic rate (the number of calories your body burns when at rest). These processes help to keep glucose levels lower after carbohydrate-rich meals.

Alongside these lifestyle changes, insulin resistance can be further addressed by replacing any nutrient deficiencies, minimizing toxic exposures, addressing gut dysbiosis and systemic inflammation, fixing HPA axis dysfunction, and the use of certain drugs and supplements, such as metformin and berberine.

## Calculate Caloric Needs Based on Your Weight Goals

Together, your choice of foods and drinks and the quantity you consume are the biggest factor in reaching your weight goals, whether it's to gain weight, lose weight or maintain weight. Discuss what your weight goal should be with your health care team, as it may need to be customized to your health and medical conditions. Never lose sight of nutrient density (choosing foods with the highest amount of nutrients per serving). Many people become depleted of nutrients when they follow restrictive diets (e.g., ketogenic, vegan, etc.) if they're not careful.

Once you know your weight goal, you'll want to find out how many calories you should be consuming each day.

My favorite calorie assessment tool is the Body Weight Planner (*www.niddk.nih.gov/bwp*) from the National Institute of Health's National Institutes of Diabetes and Digestive and Kidney Diseases. You input your weight, sex, age, height, physical activity level, goal weight, how long you want to take to reach your goal weight, and whether you intend to change your physical activity level during your weight loss, and it calculates for you the caloric requirements to either maintain your current weight or reach a gain or loss goal within your desired timeframe. An example of this assessment is shown in this next figure.

# Calculate Your Optimal Caloric Intake to Achieve a Desired Body Weight: NIH Body Weight Planner

U.S. Department of Health and Human Services

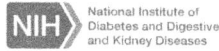

**NIH** National Institute of
Diabetes and Digestive
and Kidney Diseases

## Body Weight Planner

| Balancing Your Food and Activity

Step 1 of 4 - Enter your starting information

Starting Information

| U.S. Units | Metric Units | |
|---|---|---|
| Weight | 160 | lbs |
| Sex | Male | |
| Age | 49 | yrs |
| Height | 5 ft 9 in | |
| Physical Activity Level | 1.6 | Estimate Your Level |

## Body Weight Planner | Balancing Your Food and Activity

Goal Weight    Lifestyle Change

**Weight Goal**

| Goal Weight | 160 | lbs |
|---|---|---|
| I want to reach my goal in | 90 | days |

OR select a date

| I want to reach my goal by | 7/15/2023 | |

**Physical Activity Change (Optional)**

**Weight Change Phase**

| To reach my goal, I will change my physical activity by | 0 Calculate | % |

**Goal Maintenance Phase**

| To maintain my goal, I will change my physical activity by | 0 Calculate | % |

→ Results

| Calories | Kilojoules |
|---|---|
| In order to *maintain* your current weight, you should eat: | **2,535** Calories/day |
| To *reach* your goal of **155 lbs** in **90 days**, you should eat: | **2,322** Calories/day |
| To *maintain* your goal of **155 lbs**, you should eat: | **2,477** Calories/day |

## Tracking Your Calories

Rest assured, you do not need to track calories indefinitely, but I do highly recommend using a calorie tracking app on your mobile phone or other electronic device for at least the first few months to track your food intake. My favorite is Cronometer (*cronometer.com*). This online tracking tool is very helpful for you when optimizing your nutrient intake as well. (We'll talk about this more in this chapter's section on nutrient deficiencies.) You can use calorie and nutrient-tracking apps while consulting with a registered dietician or nutritionist too, as they help to guide you to improve your caloric intake and the nutrient density in your diet.

If your goal is to lose body fat, I recommend the Data Driven Fasting (DDF) online course, as I mentioned on page 25 at *www.datadrivenfasting.com/home*. DDF utilizes blood sugar testing (either via a finger stick or continuous glucose monitor) to guide an intermittent fasting approach that is proven to healthfully lower fasting glucose, insulin, and body fat levels over time. We know that in order to burn body fat, we need to first burn off much of the glucose circulating in the body and then deplete liver glycogen and free fatty acids in the blood.

As advocated in the DDF program, one of the most successful and sustainable fat loss approaches combines blood sugar-informed intermittent fasting and following a nutrient-dense, higher protein, lower glycemic diet. Studies show that, in the vast majority of individuals, as the percentage of protein increases in their diet, their satiety (feeling satisfied, not hungry) signals increase and caloric intake decreases.

I typically recommend limiting net carbohydrates (defined as grams of total carbohydrates minus grams of dietary fiber minus grams of sugar alcohol) to less than 50 grams per day in my patients with insulin resistance, although some may find success with lower or higher net carbohydrate limits. You can assess your response to varying amounts of net carbohydrates using blood sugar testing and tracking (diet, body composition, and weight) over time. The DDF program helps guide you on how to do this efficiently and effectively.

## Are You Overweight?

As mentioned earlier, one of the first steps that I recommend to my patients is that we determine whether or not they are overweight, underweight, or at their ideal body weight. There are many methods to assess what your ideal body weight is. If this section feels rather detailed, it's because I think it is important to explain the different methods necessary to determine whether you have insulin resistance and the various ways how to measure your body's composition to determine your ideal body weight using the different tools available.

### Calculate Your Ideal Body Weight

**Calculator. net**

- Males:    Use "Devine" formula
- Females: Use "Robinson" formula

home / fitness & health / ideal weight calculator

#### Ideal Weight Calculator

The *Ideal Weight Calculator* computes ideal body weight (IBW) ranges based on height, gender, and age. The idea of finding the IBW using a formula has been sought after by many experts for a long time. Currently, there persist several popular formulas, and our Ideal Weight Calculator provides their results for side-to-side comparisons.

Modify the values and click the Calculate button to use

| US Units | Metric Units | Other Units |
| --- | --- | --- |

Age    70    ages 2 - 80

Gender  ● male  ○ female

Height  5   feet   9   inches

Calculate ▶  Clear

**Result**

The ideal weight based on popular formulas:

| Formula | Ideal Weight |
| --- | --- |
| Robinson (1983) | 152.3 lbs | ← |
| Miller (1983) | 151.9 lbs |
| Devine (1974) | 155.9 lbs | ← |
| Hamwi (1964) | 159.4 lbs |
| Healthy BMI Range | 125.3 - 169.3lbs |

https://www.calculator.net/ideal-weight-calculator.html

I like to use an ideal body weight calculator, such as this one from calculator.net (*www.calculator.net/ideal-weight-calculator.html*). It's recommended that males use the Devine formula and females use the Robinson formula to assess their ideal body weight. The figure above shows that a 70-year-old male who is five feet nine inches tall has an ideal body weight of 155.9 pounds, using the Devine formula.

## What's Your Body Fat Percentage?

There are many methods to determine your body fat. For example, it can be determined through visual graphics. The next figure features male and female models and their body fat percentage ranges.

### Ideal Body Weight Percentages

| Description | Women | Men |
|---|---|---|
| Essential fat | 10–13% | 2–5% |
| Athletes | 14–20% | 6–13% |
| Fitness | 21–24% | 14–17% |
| Average | 25–31% | 18–25% |
| Obese | 32+% | 25+% |

The Navy body fat calculator (*www.calculator.net/body-fat-calculator.html*) is another tool to reasonably estimate one's body fat percentage using an individual's age, sex, height, neck circumference, and waist circumference. This next figure shows a sample calculation for a 50-year-old male who is five feet nine inches tall.

## Calculate Your Body Fat:
## Navy Body Fat Calculator

| | |
|---|---|
| Age | 50 years |
| Sex | male ▾ |
| Height | 5 ft▾ 9 in▾ |
| Neck circumference | 15 in▾ |
| Waist circumference | 33 in▾ |
| Body fat | 15.9 % |

Congratulations! You meet the US Navy body fat standards!

Bioelectrical impedance digital scales can also be used; however, the accuracy will vary based on your hydration status (accuracy plus or minus 5–10%). These scales are very useful for tracking trends over time, even if they aren't the most precise measurement of body fat percentage.

My personal favorite method to more accurately assess body fat percentage is with a DEXA (dual-energy X-ray absorptiometry) scan. Most DEXA scans are used to determine someone's bone density to find out if they have normal bone density or lower bone density (osteopenia or osteoporosis), but some can also assess body fat and muscle mass. DEXA scans are the most accurate of the methods mentioned above to determine body composition.

There are other methods to measure body fat that may also be helpful:
- Displacement methods (hydrostatic underwater weighing, "BOD POD")
- 3-D body scans
- CT scan
- MRI

## Alternative Assessments for Body Fat

Calculating body mass index (see *www.calculator.net/bmi-calculator.html* and *www.omnicalculator.com/health/bmi*) is often done in medical practices as a surrogate measurement for a patient's body fat. BMI is calculated with online calculators using age, gender, height, and weight. While BMI may not be the best assessment tool for determining how overweight, underweight, or of normal weight a person is, years of research have correlated increased BMI with many chronic health conditions, including but not limited to type 2 diabetes, cardiovascular disease, and cancer.

Increasingly, studies show that a better assessment of somebody's body fat is their waist–height ratio (see *www.omnicalculator.com/health/waist-height-ratio*). The waist–height ratio is a measure of the distribution of body fat (specifically, their central or visceral fat), and correlates more closely than BMI with most health outcomes. The preponderance of data indicates that a waist–height ratio of 0.5 or greater is associated with worse health outcomes and shortened lifespan.[5]

# Nutrient Deficiencies

Have you ever wondered if you are eating enough nutrients to ensure that you do not have any nutrient deficiencies? I test many of my cancer patients and survivors using NutrEval (a high-quality nutrient test), and the results indicate that the vast majority have multiple nutrient deficiencies. Whether this is a result of nutrient-poor foods, food selection, nutrient-absorption problems, increased demands on the body,

---

[5]   Margaret Ashwell, et al., "Waist-to-height ratio is more predictive of years of life lost than body mass index," PLoS One, 2014 Sep 8;9(9):e103483, https://pubmed.ncbi.nlm.nih.gov/25198730.

or a combination of two or more, we want to know where you stand on your nutrient status during and after your cancer treatments.

Unfortunately, most physicians do not perform nutritional assessments on their patients. That means you may be deficient in many nutrients without anyone knowing it, and these deficiencies can influence your overall health, immune function, systemic inflammation, insulin resistance, cancer outcomes and quality of life. If we can determine your specific deficiencies, then we can make recommendations for the specific nutrients you need to take to fill these gaps.

As you can see in the next figure, I find that the majority of my patients have low nutrient levels—there are widespread deficiencies across multiple vitamins, minerals, amino acids, and omega-3 fatty acids. It's particularly shocking to see that 83% of my patients had deficiencies in multiple amino acids, the building blocks for protein. Numerous B vitamin deficiencies, as well as low levels of crucial antioxidants (such as glutathione and alpha lipoic acid/ALA) were also prolific.

## Nutrient Deficiencies Are Very Common in Cancer Patients: Percentages of Initial Nutrient Deficiencies in Dr. Lawenda's Cancer Patients (73 patients)

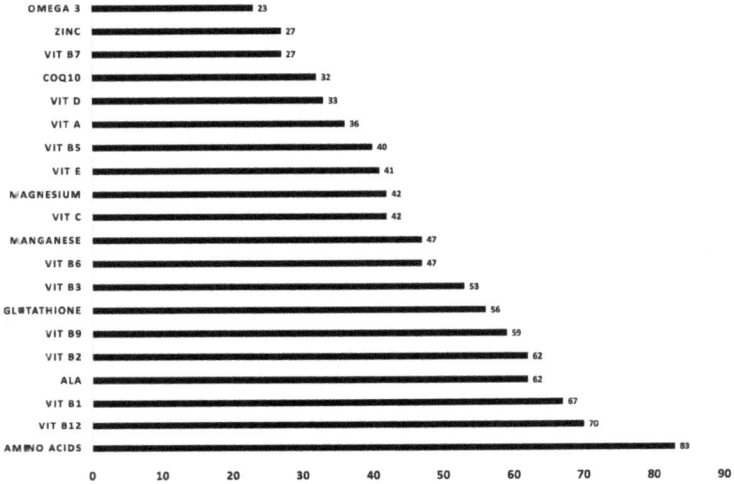

| Nutrient | Percentage |
|---|---|
| OMEGA 3 | 23 |
| ZINC | 27 |
| VIT B7 | 27 |
| COQ10 | 32 |
| VIT D | 33 |
| VIT A | 36 |
| VIT B5 | 40 |
| VIT E | 41 |
| MAGNESIUM | 42 |
| VIT C | 42 |
| MANGANESE | 47 |
| VIT B6 | 47 |
| VIT B3 | 53 |
| GLUTATHIONE | 56 |
| VIT B9 | 59 |
| VIT B2 | 62 |
| ALA | 62 |
| VIT B1 | 67 |
| VIT B12 | 70 |
| AMINO ACIDS | 83 |

Nutrient deficiencies are associated with various symptoms and pathophysiological health states, as shown in this next figure. We know that having adequate levels of all vitamins, minerals, amino acids, and fatty acids is essential to support a healthy immune system and minimize systemic inflammation.

## Contributors to and Indirect Effects of Nutrient Deficiencies on Cancer Development, Growth, Metastasis and Recurrence

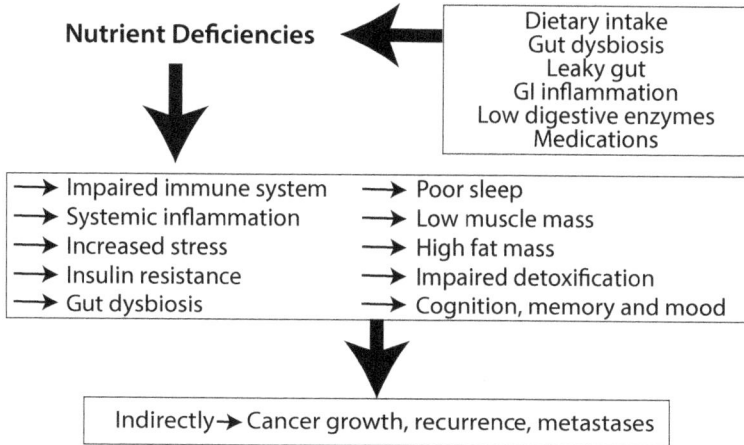

**Nutrient Deficiencies** ← Dietary intake
Gut dysbiosis
Leaky gut
GI inflammation
Low digestive enzymes
Medications

→ Impaired immune system   → Poor sleep
→ Systemic inflammation   → Low muscle mass
→ Increased stress   → High fat mass
→ Insulin resistance   → Impaired detoxification
→ Gut dysbiosis   → Cognition, memory and mood

Indirectly→ Cancer growth, recurrence, metastases

Nutrients, such as vitamins, minerals, amino acids and fatty acids, are what we call "co-factors," which means they are needed by the body to perform important processes. These nutrients are involved in most enzymatic reactions and cellular processes throughout the body, so when we have deficiencies, these can cause our cancer- and infection-fighting white blood cells not to work optimally, our tissues to be more susceptible to injury and free radical damage, reduce our ability to detoxify, impair insulin receptor function, decrease ability to maintain or grow muscle mass, cause mitochondrial dysfunction, and more.

Many nutrient deficiencies have been associated with an increased risk for cancer development, progression, and mortality. These include:
- Vitamins A, B3, B6, B9, B12, C, D, K
- Minerals, such as zinc and selenium
- Protein

Many nutrients play important roles in mitochondrial energy production and detoxification, gene regulation and methylation. And while specific nutrient deficiencies may not directly correlate to worse cancer outcomes, the indirect associations from their related pathophysiological states (e.g., insulin resistance, systemic inflammation, impaired immune function, decreased methylation activity, and impaired mitochondrial energy production) are often highly associated with increased cancer growth, recurrence, and metastatic rates.

For example, numerous vitamin deficiencies have been linked to insulin resistance, which can promote tumor growth. Various nutrient deficiencies can also lead to impaired immune function, mitochondrial energy production, and methylation activity, as illustrated in the next two figures, and also lead to increased tumor growth through the production of pro-inflammatory cytokines.

### Examples of Nutrients Involved in Optimizing Immune Health

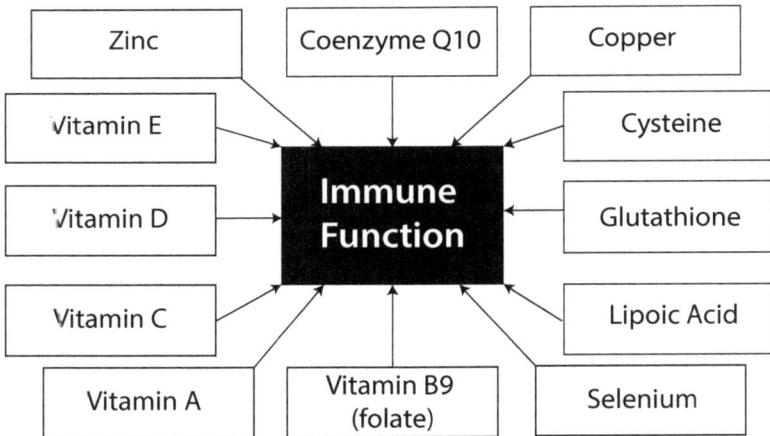

| Zinc | Coenzyme Q10 | Copper |
|---|---|---|
| Vitamin E | | Cysteine |
| Vitamin D | **Immune Function** | Glutathione |
| Vitamin C | | Lipoic Acid |
| Vitamin A | Vitamin B9 (folate) | Selenium |

Studies show that these compounds support immune function. It's important to first measure one's nutrient levels before taking supplements.

## Examples of Nutrients Involved in
## Optimizing Insulin Sensitivity

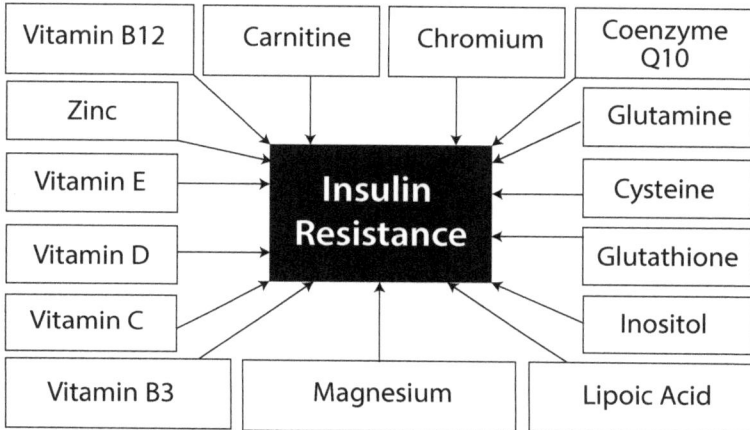

| | | | |
|---|---|---|---|
| Vitamin B12 | Carnitine | Chromium | Coenzyme Q10 |
| Zinc | | | Glutamine |
| Vitamin E | **Insulin Resistance** | | Cysteine |
| Vitamin D | | | Glutathione |
| Vitamin C | | | Inositol |
| Vitamin B3 | Magnesium | | Lipoic Acid |

Studies show that these compounds support insulin sensitivity, insulin secretion, and deficiencies and complications common in those with insulin resistance function.

## Assessing and Addressing Nutrient Deficiencies

Nutrient assessment, as shown on the next page, can be done through lab testing, such as the NutrEval test I mentioned earlier or through food tracking software such as Cronometer (the software with the most complete nutrient profiles of foods).

## Nutrient Testing: (Genova Diagnostics, NutrEval Sample Report)

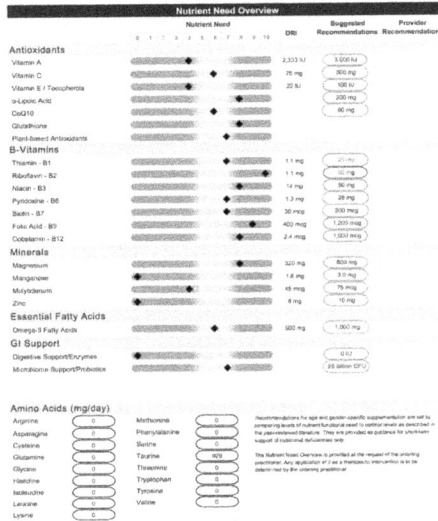

Once deficiencies have been identified, these can be addressed in a number of ways. It is possible to work with a dietitian or nutritionist to improve your diet and make sure you are getting all of the nutrients you need from whole food sources. Additionally, you can consult an integrative or functional medicine provider who is qualified to recommend supplements that will help fill any nutritional gaps in your diet.

I often recommend taking a DIY approach with online tools, such as Optimising Nutrition's Micronutrient (*optimisingnutrition.com/micros-masterclass*) and Macronutrient (*optimisingnutrition.com/macros-masterclass*) courses, to guide you on how to improve your diet and address nutrient deficiencies without using supplements. Additionally, I collaborated with Optimising Nutrition on the development of three recipe books for cancer patients (see *optimisingnutrition.com/nutrient-dense-foods-meals-cancer/#h-the-recipe-books*) that focus on nutrient-dense diets for everyone, whether you need to gain weight, lose weight, or maintain your optimal weight.

Since protein is the most common deficiency I find in my patients, let's take a quick look at a simple way to determine how much protein to consume per day.

Step 1: Using a calculator, such as the one at *www.calculator.net/ideal-weight-calculator.html*, get an estimate of your ideal body weight. (Males: use the Devine formula; females: use the Robinson formula)

Step 2: Convert your ideal body weight estimate from pounds to kilograms (dividing the number of pounds by 2.2 will give you your weight in kilograms)

Step 3: Select your protein multiplier (grams of protein to consume per day per kilogram of ideal body weight):

- ◦ 1.4–1.8 (Sedentary and healthy weight, maintain muscle)
- ◦ 1.6–2.0 (Active and healthy weight, maintain muscle)
- ◦ 1.6–3.2 (Active and want to build muscle and lose body fat)

Step 4: Calculate your total daily protein (the grams of protein you should ingest per day is your ideal body weight in kilograms times your protein multiplier—an ounce equals about 28.5 grams)

Step 5: To optimize your body's use of this protein, spread it as evenly as possible across each of your meals.

Another excellent tool to help you calculate your protein requirements (as well as calories, fat and carbohydrates) to achieve your weight goals is the Optimising Nutrition Macro Calculator, *optimisingnutrition.com/macro-calculator*.

I recommend that anyone who has previously been found to have low nutrient levels get a follow-up assessment (either with a NutrEval test or tracking dietary intake with Cronometer) to determine if the interventions you made have been successful.

If you continue to experience nutrient deficiencies, I recommend getting a gut health test, such as the GI MAP test. This tests for issues related to the gut, such as dysbiosis (imbalance in your microbiome), leaky gut (where your intestinal wall is overly permeable, enabling both the loss of nutrients into your stool and enabling fecal organisms and chemicals to "leak" into your body and cause low grade systemic inflammation), intestinal inflammation and immune activity, digestive enzyme adequacy, and gluten sensitivity. Each of these issues can decrease your body's ability to absorb nutrients, thereby contributing to nutrient deficiencies.

It is essential to work with a functional medicine provider who can help you interpret your results and provide guidance on how to address any persistent areas of concern. I often recommend also working with a dietitian or nutritionist, especially when multiple deficiencies are identified.

# Chronic Stress

Stress is something most of us can relate to. Even if we don't feel like we're in a constant state of stress, we've all experienced stressful situations before. This can stem from many different sources, including work and school deadlines, interpersonal conflicts, or even just feeling overwhelmed by the number of things we have to get done in a day.

While it's true that not all stress is bad for you—some forms of stress can actually be beneficial—it's important to recognize that chronic stress is harmful and can cause long-lasting damage, if not managed correctly. In order to understand why some types of stress are more harmful than others, we must first understand what exactly happens in our bodies when we experience stress.

There's an important distinction between acute and chronic stress. Acute stress usually is due to some instigating factor that comes and goes over a short period of time. Individuals who experience acute stress usually recover from it shortly after the stressor has been dealt with or mitigated. Chronic stress, on the other hand, occurs when a stressor continues to exert its effects on an individual over months, or possibly years. It is chronic stress that exerts long-lasting negative effects throughout the body. These effects are promulgated by stress hormone-signaling molecules that are produced primarily in the adrenal glands, including epinephrine, norepinephrine, and cortisol.

Exposure to these stress hormones can be beneficial when they activate fight or flight responses designed to help protect against infections and facilitate wound healing. However, chronically elevated or even low levels of these hormones (mainly cortisol) can lead to insulin resistance, chronic inflammation, hypertension, immune suppression, and cardiovascular disease. Chronic stress can also impair anticancer immune activity and indirectly promote cancer progression through numerous mechanisms.

Studies also demonstrate that chronically elevated stress hormone levels can cause changes to our genes (i.e., turning off anti-cancer genes and increasing tumor growth factor genes) that may have a significant impact on the development and growth of cancer.

# Stress: Internal and External, Real and Perceived

**HPA Axis Influencers:**

→ Lifestyle (mental stress, exercise, diet, sleep, toxins)

→ Blood sugar regulation

→ Systemic inflammation

→ Oxidative stress

→ Mitochondrial health

**Chronically High or Low Cortisol Can Lead to:**

→ Insulin resistance

→ Weight (fat) gain

→ Immune suppression

→ Chronic fatigue

→ Gut dysbiosis, leaky gut

→ Hypertension

→ Low muscle mass and bone density

→ Sleep problems (low melatonin)

→ Neurocognitive/mood problems

→ Eventual low cortisol levels due to negative feedback on HPA axis

→ Impaired NK cell activity, systemic inflammation

# Stress: Internal and External, Real and Perceived (continued)

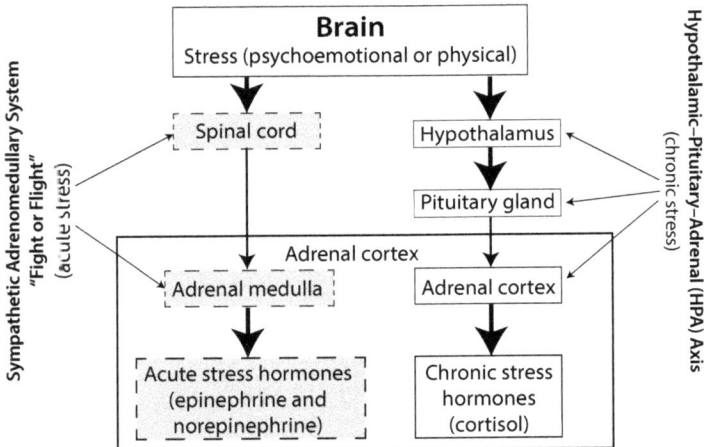

**Brain**
Stress (psychoemotional or physical)

Sympathetic Adrenomedullary System "Fight or Flight" (acute stress)

Hypothalamic–Pituitary–Adrenal (HPA) Axis (chronic stress)

Spinal cord

Hypothalamus

Pituitary gland

Adrenal cortex

Adrenal medulla

Adrenal cortex

Acute stress hormones (epinephrine and norepinephrine)

Chronic stress hormones (cortisol)

Once a tumor has developed, chronic stress may also affect numerous mechanisms that can potentially lead to cancer progression. Stress hormones:

- increase tumor growth through stimulation of beta-adrenergic receptors
- increase tumor cell invasiveness and metastatic activity
- increase tumor blood-vessel growth rates
- suppress natural killer (NK) cell activity (immune suppression)
- reduce the cancer-killing effects of chemotherapy

In a meta-analysis of 165 studies of chronic stress and cancer outcomes,[6] chronic stress was associated with up to 21% higher risk of developing cancer and 133% higher risk of dying from cancer.

## Deleterious Effects of Stress on the Body and Lifestyle Habits

→ Neurocognitive Impairments    → Low Muscle Mass

→ Cardiovascular Disease    → High Visceral Fat Mass

→ Gut Dysbiosis    → Insulin Resistance

→ Chronic Stress    → Nutrient Deficiencies

→ Inadequate or Excessive Sleep    → Poor Diet/Nutrient Deficiencies

"Cancer and stress: NextGen strategies," Brain, Behavior, and Immunity, Vol. 93, March 2021, pp. 368–83

When the brain processes stress, it does so through communication from multiple areas, including the amygdala, hippocampus, and prefrontal cortex. These signals converge

---

6   Chida, Yoichi, Hamer, Wardle, Steptoe, "Do stress-related psychosocial factors contribute to cancer incidence and survival?" Nat Clin Pract Oncol., 2008 Aug;5(8):466-75, doi: 10.1038/ncponc1134, Epub 2008 May 20, https://pubmed.ncbi.nlm.nih.gov/18493231.

at a structure called the hypothalamus and lead to the release of CRH (corticotropin-releasing hormone), which then signals the pituitary gland to release ACTH (adrenocorticotropic hormone). ACTH circulates through the blood until it reaches the adrenal gland, where it causes the release of norepinephrine, epinephrine, and cortisol. This is the HPA axis—the hypothalamus–pituitary–adrenal axis—that I mentioned earlier in this chapter, in the section on immune function.

The regulation of this system is under tight hormonal control and feedback, but it can be disrupted by chronic stress and many other factors, such as inadequate or excessive sleep or exercise, low muscle mass, high visceral fat mass, insulin resistance, nutrient deficiencies, toxic chemicals, gut dysbiosis and leaky gut, and systemic inflammation. This can lead to a condition called HPA axis dysfunction, which can have widespread deleterious effects on your health.

## Assessing Stress, HPA Axis Dysfunction, and Melatonin

### A Functional Medicine Approach to Optimize HPA Axis Function

High or Low Cortisol
(HPA axis dysfunction)

Dark Gray boxes: Assess chronic stress with HPA axis testing (DUTCH Test) and/or heart rate variability (HRV) tracking.

| DUTCH Test | HRV Tracking |
|---|---|

Medium Gray boxes: If chronic stress is an issue:

| Stress Management | Minimize Body Fat | Supportive Supplements |
|---|---|---|
| Exercise | Increase Muscle Mass | Sleep |

Light Gray boxes: Consider any of the many stress management recommendations listed in the figure above, if any of these conditions are identified:

| Systemic Inflammation | Nutrient Deficiencies |
|---|---|

| Dysbiosis/Leaky Gut/GI Inflammation/Food Sensitivities | |
|---|---|

Most oncology practices assess for stress using risk assessment questionnaires, such as the NCCN Distress Thermometer (*www.nccn.org/docs/default-source/patient-resources/nccn_distress_thermometer.pdf*). This questionnaire incorporates a spectrum of concerns: physical, emotional, social, practical, and spiritual or religious; and the patient indicates their level of distress on a scale from zero to 10, where 10 is extreme distress and zero is no distress. Note that "distress" is the term used in place of "stress," so as to encompass both psychoemotional issues, like stress, anxiety, or depression, and physical issues.

To measure HPA axis dysfunction (impacted by chronic or long-term stress), we use cortisol testing (such as the DUTCH test) throughout the day and evening via saliva and urine tests. HPA axis dysfunction is diagnosed when one's cortisol levels are either higher or lower than the standard range.

Heart rate variability (HRV) tracking is another way to assess one's state of stress. The *greater* your heart rate variability, meaning the more beat-to-beat variations in your heart rate, the *less* stressed you are. Think of it as your heart exhibiting greater flexibility in coping with stress signals from your nervous system. The lower your HRV, meaning the less beat-to-beat variation there is in your heartbeats, the more stressed you are. Stress, particularly chronic stress, decreases the beat-to-beat variations (lower HRV) in one's heart rate. We all want to see our HRV go up over time.

HRV is measured by recording the time interval between one heartbeat and the next, over time. It is best measured at night while asleep, but it can also be measured when at rest while awake. There are no well-established optimal HRV ranges. Instead, HRV is unique for each individual. When tracking your HRV, you simply want to see improvements (increasing HRV) over time. There are many devices on the market that measure HRV. My favorite for tracking HRV while asleep is the Oura ring. Another device, Inner Balance (by HeartMath), is my preferred device to assess and give real-time feedback on one's HRV during paced breathing exercises (biofeedback). Instead of quantifying HRV, this device uses a visual alternative called heart "coherence" that you can watch on an app on your smartphone.

Importantly, studies have found that having a higher HRV correlates with better survival outcomes across many cancer types.

In order for the human body to properly regulate the sleep–wake cycle, it must maintain a certain amount of melatonin at night. Melatonin is a hormone produced by the brain's pineal gland and is responsible for regulating sleep–wake cycles. Unfortunately, in people with HPA axis dysfunction, the pineal gland often cannot create adequate amounts of melatonin. (The HPA axis controls the release of stress hormones from the adrenal glands.) When the stress hormone cortisol is too high at night, this suppresses the pineal gland's production of melatonin. Having higher nighttime cortisol levels can therefore make it difficult for you to fall asleep and/or stay asleep.

We always want to have low nighttime cortisol levels to facilitate melatonin release and better sleep. (Getting adequate, high-quality sleep is essential for optimal health.)

The DUTCH test assesses both cortisol and melatonin levels. If we identify low levels of melatonin and/or high levels of evening cortisol, we can address this in several ways: optimizing sleep, stress management, exercise, and possibly dietary supplementation (such as certain botanical/adaptogenic compounds, melatonin, micronutrients). Additionally, nutrient and systemic inflammatory marker testing can be assessed, as nutrient deficiencies and chronic systemic inflammation also contribute to HPA axis dysfunction.

## A Functional Medicine Approach to Optimize Melatonin Levels
### Low Melatonin

Dark Gray boxes: Assess melatonin level with the DUTCH test.

| DUTCH Test | |
|---|---|

Medium Gray boxes: If low melatonin level, consider these interventions:

| Stress Management | Supportive Supplements, Nutrients or Drugs |
|---|---|
| Exercise | Sleep Hygiene |

Light Gray boxes: Consider additional functional medicine testing to assess for other contributing factors:

| Systemic Inflammation | Nutrients |
|---|---|
| High Cortisol (HPA axis dysfunction) | |

## Stress Reduction

It's been well established through countless studies that stress reduction education, programs, and interventions are effective in mitigating chronic stress and improving numerous physiological parameters and health conditions. While some skepticism remains concerning the potential benefits for stress reduction to improve cancer outcomes, substantial evidence supports that there is a link between chronic stress, the immune system, systemic inflammation, and cancer.

## After relaxation training and stress-minimizing advice, breast cancer patients had a 45% lower risk of cancer recurring and 56% reduced cancer mortality

Many preclinical studies in animals have demonstrated reductions in cancer progression and metastases with interventions that minimize either stress or neurohormonal signaling by blocking beta-adrenergic receptors (stress hormone receptors).

Stress has been shown to increase the risk of developing metastatic cancer in mice. In a study[7] examining this relationship, researchers found that stressed mice were up to 30 times more likely than the mice in the control group to develop metastases after injection with breast cancer cells. These results suggest that stress may be a contributing factor in the spread of cancer. The authors also found that stress hormones may play a role in cancer progression, as immune system cells in stressed mice were found to be impaired by the activity of stress hormones, increasing the ability of the injected cancer cells to gain access to the blood system and spread.

Interestingly, when the researchers tested the effects of a stress hormone blocker (propranolol, a non-selective beta-blocking blood pressure drug) on the stressed mice, the negative effects of the stress hormones were completely blocked. This led the researchers to conclude that propranolol, which is an inexpensive and widely available blood pressure medication, could play a future role in helping to reduce the

---

7   Sloan, Erika K., et al., "The Sympathetic Nervous System Induces a Metastatic Switch in Primary Breast Cancer," Cancer Research, Vol. 70, Issue 18, 15 September 2010, http://cancerres.aacrjournals.org/content/70/18/7042.

risk of cancer progression. Numerous studies have reported improved cancer outcomes in cancer patients who take non-selective beta-blocking drugs. While further research is needed to better understand how stress hormones affect cancer progression, these findings are important, because they suggest that reducing or blocking stress hormones may be an important tool in preventing the progression of cancer.

One of my favorite clinical studies[8] found that breast cancer patients who received relaxation training and advice on minimizing stress had a 45% reduced risk of cancer recurrence and a 56% reduction in cancer mortality! Additionally, the study found that patients in the intervention group, the ones given tools to minimize stress, had improvements in multiple immune function measurements and quality of life outcomes. These findings suggest that psychological interventions may be an effective way to improve outcomes for cancer patients.

The study's authors suggest that the mechanism for this improvement is due to the positive effects of stress reduction on the immune system. Stress has been shown to have a negative impact on immunity, and it is possible that by reducing stress, the intervention group was able to improve their immunity and reduce their risk of cancer recurrence. Additionally, the relaxation techniques used in the intervention may have helped to reduce systemic inflammation, which has also been linked to an increased risk of cancer and worse cancer outcomes.

Psychological interventions can play an important role in cancer care and treatment. Relaxation techniques and stress management should be considered as part of a comprehensive treatment plan for any cancer patient and survivor. Notably, reducing or blocking stress hormones (through lifestyle modifications and/or medications and supplements) may eventually be confirmed in future studies as potential new avenues for improving cancer outcomes.

---

8   Barbara Andersen, et al., "Psychologic Intervention Improves Survival in Breast Cancer Patients. A Randomized Clinical Trial," *Cancer*, 15 Dec 2008, https://pubmed.ncbi.nlm.nih.gov/19016270.

## My Favorite Stress Reduction Approaches

Make sure to schedule some time each day for a dedicated stress reduction activity. This could be something as simple as meditation, paced breathing, or biofeedback. Just one session of these activities can improve your mood and reduce stress levels. However, to see more lasting effects, it's important to make stress reduction a regular part of your routine. Think of it like taking medication: you need to do it every day to see the benefits. So, commit to incorporating regular stress reduction activities into your daily schedule, and you'll reap the many benefits of lower stress levels and a better mood.

I am always on the lookout for effective tools that can help my patients reduce the effects of stress on their bodies and minds. Here are some of my favorites.

**Meditation** – This can actually change the neuronal structure and connections in your brain. Studies have found that after just eight weeks of 10–20 minutes of meditation, three times a week, you can see an increase in the brain's grey matter density responsible for emotional regulation, planning, and problem solving. Additionally, the brain's cortical matter volume increases, which impacts our learning and memory processing. The amygdala also shrinks—this is the center of our brain that is in charge of *how* we feel stress, fear, and anxiety. When these changes occur in the brain, they result in decreased sympathetic nervous system (the 'fight or flight' or stress part of the nervous system) activity and increased parasympathetic nervous system (responsible for relaxation) activity, as well as decreased activation of the HPA axis and lower levels of stress hormones like cortisol. There are many different types of meditation practices, but they all share certain key features that have been shown to be beneficial for reducing mental stress and improving overall well-being. Some of my favorite online meditation apps include 10 Percent Happier (*www.tenpercent.com*), Calm (*www.calm.com*), and

Headspace (*www.headspace.com / meditation / sleep*). I highly recommend giving them a try if you're looking to add meditation into your life in a simple and convenient way.

**Biofeedback** – This is a powerful and effective tool to reduce stress and improve overall health. By tracking your stress levels through physiological indicators, such as heart rate variability, biofeedback allows you to visualize the results of your efforts to reduce stress and increase relaxation. One of the best biofeedback devices on the market is Inner Balance. The device is easy to use: simply wear the ear clip heart rhythm sensor, which wirelessly sends real-time heartbeat rhythm (a variation on heart rate variability called "coherence") readings to a free downloadable app on your smartphone (*store.heartmath.com / inner-balance*). As you relax, the app shows you how well you are doing. With regular practice, you can learn to control your body's response to stressors and improve your overall health and wellbeing. Why not give it a try? You may be surprised at just how effective biofeedback can be.

**Paced breathing** – My personal favorite is "4–7–8 breathing", a simple and powerful relaxation technique that can be done anywhere and at any time when you are feeling stressed. This technique is based on a yoga practice called *pranayama*, which was popularized by Dr. Andrew Weil and many other health experts. Start by sitting or standing comfortably with your back straight and your shoulders relaxed. Next, take a deep breath in through your nose, counting slowly to four as you inhale. Hold your breath for a count of seven, then exhale slowly through your mouth for a count of eight. Continue this cycle of deep breathing for several minutes, focusing on the gentle in and out movements of your belly as you breathe. Paced breathing is a highly effective way to reduce stress and achieve a sense of calmness and relaxation. It can be done anywhere, at any time, and requires very little effort or concentration. If you are feeling stressed or anxious, try using paced breathing to help regain your sense of inner peace and calmness. With regular practice, this simple technique can help you manage stress more effectively in your everyday life.

**Sauna** – Sauna use is a great way to reduce stress. There are different types of saunas, but we don't know if one is more effective than the other. Traditional saunas heat up the air to about 185°F, while infrared saunas only reach about 140°F. Infrared rays penetrate more deeply into the body, which means you start sweating at a lower temperature than in a traditional sauna, allowing you to enjoy a longer session without overheating. The physiological effects of sauna use are well documented, and include increases in HRV and parasympathetic (relaxation) response from the body's autonomic nervous system. Additionally, sauna use has been shown to have a variety of other beneficial effects for cancer patients and for overall health, including improved circulation, increased immune function, detoxification and decreased systemic inflammation. Whether used alone or as part of a broader treatment approach, incorporating regular sauna sessions into your routine can be an effective way to promote overall wellness and improve your physical and mental health.

## Other Effective Stress Reduction Approaches

- Acupuncture
- Yoga
- Guided imagery
- Supplements & botanical compounds
- Exercise
- Getting quality sleep

- Professional mental health counseling – Ask your health care provider for a referral. There are also remote telehealth counseling services that make counseling much more convenient, such as Ginger (*www.ginger.com*) and Talkspace (*www.talkspace.com*).

# Gut Health

Our gut health is critical to our overall health and well-being. A healthy gut is necessary for a strong immune system, preventing inflammation in the body and even for immunotherapy drugs to be effective. Our gut microorganisms help in digestion, absorption, and creation of micronutrients, toxin breakdown and elimination, production of hormones that improve mental health and mood, and to reduce systemic inflammation and improve insulin sensitivity.

There are a number of causative factors that can impact the health of the gut, including diet, imbalance of intestinal microorganisms (dysbiosis), food sensitivities, drugs/medications, chemicals, radiation, sleep problems, and stress. These factors can influence the development or progression of many pathophysiological states, such as an impaired immune system, increased systemic inflammation, HPA axis dysfunction, and/or insulin resistance. While these conditions do not always correlate with an increased risk of cancer development, progression, or recurrence, many are indirectly associated.

## Indirect Effects of Gut Health on Cancer Development, Growth, Metastasis and Recurrence

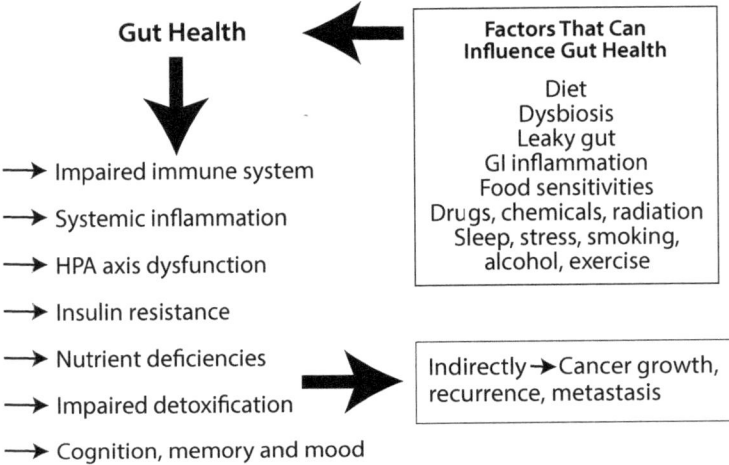

**Gut Health**  ⬅️  | Factors That Can Influence Gut Health |

⬇️

→ Impaired immune system

→ Systemic inflammation

→ HPA axis dysfunction

→ Insulin resistance

→ Nutrient deficiencies

→ Impaired detoxification

→ Cognition, memory and mood

**Factors That Can Influence Gut Health**

Diet
Dysbiosis
Leaky gut
GI inflammation
Food sensitivities
Drugs, chemicals, radiation
Sleep, stress, smoking, alcohol, exercise

➡️ Indirectly → Cancer growth, recurrence, metastasis

Examples:
- An unhealthy gut microbiota has been linked to colorectal cancer risk. Imbalances in the gut microbiota (dysbiosis) can allow pathogenic bacteria to flourish and produce toxins that damage the DNA of intestinal cells and increase inflammation, which are both risk factors for tumor development.

- Food sensitivities can cause an inflammatory response that promotes abnormal intestinal cell proliferation in the gut and dysbiosis, both of which may encourage cancer growth.

- Chronic stress has been linked to gastrointestinal cancers due to local hormonal effects on the gut immune system and microbiome, and the production of toxic metabolites that can damage cells and their DNA.

## Assessing and Addressing Gut Health

If you're looking to improve your gut health, the first thing you need to do is assess it. I recommend getting a state-of-the-art stool test that can identify dysbiosis (an imbalance between "good" and "bad" microorganisms and their diversity), leaky gut (a condition where the intestinal lining cells are unable to contain the microorganisms, chemicals, proteins, and toxins from "leaking" into the body), gut inflammation, abnormal levels of protective antibodies, food sensitivities, and adequacy of digestive enzymes.

One great option for assessing your gut health is the GI MAP test (Diagnostic Solutions Laboratory). This comprehensive stool test analyzes key markers in a simple stool sample that are associated with some of the most common issues affecting our microbiome today. By testing these markers—which include yeast, bacteria, viruses, parasites, and more—the GI MAP can give you a clearer picture of your gut health status and help you identify any areas that need improvement. If you're looking to optimize your gut health, the GI MAP test (or GI Effects Stool Profile from Genova Diagnostics) is an excellent place to start.

One of my favorite sections of the GI MAP report is the component that looks at adequacy of digestive enzymes (steatocrit, elastase-1), markers for dysbiosis (b-glucuronidase), occult blood, intestinal immune activity (secretory IgA), gluten immune reactivity (anti-gliadin IgA), intestinal inflammation (calprotectin), and leaky gut (zonulin). Your functional medicine-trained practitioner will review these results and help you address the specific aspects of intestinal health that may need to be investigated further and optimized.

Once identified, these conditions can be addressed with dietary interventions, supplements, customized probiotics (one of my favorites is Floré, by Sun Genomics), and/or other lifestyle modifications.

We know that the microbes in your gut are influenced by what you eat. One of the most important dietary factors in maintaining a healthy gut microbiome is prebiotics.

## What Are Prebiotics?

Prebiotics should not be confused with probiotics. Prebiotics are a special type of fiber that passes through the stomach and feeds the good bacteria that live in your large intestine. Dietary fibers are carbohydrates with both soluble and insoluble parts.

**Insoluble fiber** is resistant to digestion. Insoluble fiber has many benefits, including preventing constipation and possibly reducing the risk of diverticular disease.

**Soluble fibers** can be broken down by bacteria in the gut to produce active byproducts such as **short-chain fatty acids (SCFAs)**, which are associated with many of the health benefits linked to fiber.

Short-chain fatty acids, or SCFAs, are major end products of bacterial fermentation in the colon and are known to have wide-ranging impacts on health.[9] Butyrate, in particular, is important for maintaining health via:

- regulation of the immune system
- maintenance of the epithelial barrier (preventing leaky gut)
- promotion of satiety following meals
- protection against colorectal cancer, inflammatory bowel disease, diabetes, and obesity

There are three criteria for classifying a compound as prebiotic:

1. It is resistant to stomach acid and digestive enzymes, and is not absorbed in the gastrointestinal tract

---

9   Nielson T. Baxter et al., "Dynamics of Human Gut Microbiota and Short-Chain Fatty Acids in Response to Dietary Interventions with Three Fermentable Fibers," ASM Journals, Vol. 10, No. 1, 29 January 2019, https://journals.asm.org/doi/10.1128/mbio.02566-18.

2. It is fermented by intestinal bacteria
3. It selectively promotes the growth of intestinal bacteria associated with health and well-being

Many fiber components meet these requirements, but not all. Examples of prebiotics:

- Inulin (Fructo-oligosaccharide, FOS)
- Galactose (Galacto-oligosaccharide, GOS)
- Glucose (Isomalto-oligosaccharide)
- Fructose (Lactulose)
- Xylose (Xylo-oligosaccharide, XOS)
- Arabinose (AX)

Prebiotic fiber is found in many foods, primarily fruits and vegetables:

- Asparagus
- Avocado
- Banana and plantain
- Bitter greens (e.g., dandelion greens, endive, radicchio)
- Chocolate (dark), cocoa
- Coconut meat and flour
- Coffee
- Cruciferous vegetables (e.g., cabbages, broccoli, broccolini, Brussels sprouts, kale, radishes, arugula)
- Eggplant
- Jerusalem artichoke/sunchoke
- Jicama
- Honey
- Legumes (bean, lentil, chickpea)
- Onion, leek, garlic, chive
- Whole grains (e.g., oats, barley)

The Institute of Medicine currently recommends an average of 25 grams of fiber per day for women and 38 grams per day for men.[10] However, **the average American consumes a mere 15 grams per day**.

It's not easy to get enough prebiotic fiber from all these different foods, as they contain relatively small amounts of prebiotics per serving. One of the most studied of these prebiotics is inulin. Its ability to stimulate healthy bacteria and butyrate production is well documented.

I often recommend that my patients focus on getting enough *fiber* per day, rather than worry about getting enough inulin. However, for those who don't want to consume lots of fiber-rich plants each day, I recommend that they consider taking inulin as a supplement.

Based on research, five grams of inulin a day boosts the growth of the good probiotic Bifidobacterium in your gut. Eight grams or more per day helps increase calcium absorption. Getting 12 grams of inulin a day has been shown to help promote regular bowel movements.[11]

The amount of inulin we can tolerate (the side effects include bloating, cramping, and/or loose stools) seems to vary from person to person. Most people do well with up to 10 grams of inulin a day.

## Prebiotics May Cause Problems for Those with FODMAP Sensitivities

FODMAP stands for fermentable oligosaccharides, disaccharides (lactose), monosaccharides (fructose), and polyols (sorbitol and mannitol). These fermentable short-

---

10 "Dietary Reference Intakes for Energy, Carbohydrate, Fiber, Fat, Fatty Acids, Cholesterol, Protein, and Amino Acids," Consensus Study Report, 2005, http://www.nationalacademies.org/hmd/Reports/2002/Dietary-Reference-Intakes-for-Energy-Carbohydrate-Fiber-Fat-Fatty-Acids-Cholesterol-Protein-and-Amino-Acids.aspx. This report can be downloaded or read online for free.

11 Christy Brissette, "Insulin is being added to a lot of food products. And that could be bothering your stomach," *The Washington Post*, 12 June 2019, https://www.washingtonpost.com/lifestyle/wellness/what-is-inulin-and-why-is-it-showing-up-in-so-many-food-products/2019/06/11/3ee3d4be-86ec-11e9-98c1-e945a3db8fb_story.html.

chain carbohydrates (sugars) are prevalent in our diet. Often, prebiotic-rich foods contain FODMAPs.

Researchers discovered that, in some individuals, the small intestine does not absorb FODMAPs very well. They increase the amount of fluid in the bowel. They also create more gas. That's because they are easily fermented by gut bacteria. The increased fluid and gas in the bowel leads to bloating and changes in the speed in which food is digested. This results in gas, abdominal pain, and diarrhea. Eating less of these types of carbohydrates should decrease these symptoms. Examples of these types of foods are:

- dairy-based milk, yogurt, and ice cream
- wheat-based products like bread, cereal, and crackers
- legumes, like beans, soybeans, chickpeas, lentils, and peanuts
- peaches, pears, apples, and cherries

## Lab Testing for Food Intolerances

I often recommend that patients try an elimination–reintroduction diet to try to figure out how they feel when they remove certain foods from their diet. If they are very symptomatic after consuming specific foods, this approach can be quite informative and therapeutic. Food sensitivies, however, are often subtle and hard to identify, yet still be a source of gut inflammation and leaky gut. This situation can sometimes manifest with elevated inflammatory (calprotectin) and leaky gut (zonulin) proteins detected on stool testing (i.e., a GI MAP assay), without necessarily causing dysbiosis (at least, early on in this process).

To help identify these subtler food sensitivities, I often run a high-quality IgG and IgA food intolerance test (such as the Array 10–Multiple Food Immune Reactivity Screen from Cyrex Laboratories), which simultaneously assesses immune reactions to foods, raw and/or modified, food enzymes, lectins, and artificial food additives, colorings, and gums. I then have the patient temporarily (about six months) remove the foods from their diet that are identified on the test as causing a food sensitivity immune reaction, and help them address any co-existing dysbiosis and any of the other factors that may also be affecting their gut health. After excluding these foods from the diet, the gut immune system will often become less sensitive to them over time. We can then slowly reintroduce those foods and either retest in the future to assess for continued sensitivity or follow symptomatically. Sometimes the use of probiotics, digestive enzymes and other "gut healing" supplements may be recommended.

What is the difference between a food sensitivity, a food intolerance, and a food allergy? Food sensitivities, intolerances, and food allergies exist on a spectrum. They can appear in different forms, depending on the immune system's response to a particular food. On one end of the spectrum is sensitivity, which is not life-threatening but causes uncomfortable symptoms, like indigestion, and digestive issues, such as diarrhea or constipation. On the other end of the spectrum is a food allergy, which triggers a serious immune system response and can be life-threatening. However, even though food sensitivity and food intolerance are less severe than a food allergy, they can still cause inflammation in your gut and impact your immune system.

A food sensitivity and food intolerance are conditions that affect the way your body responds to certain foods. These can be caused by immune reactions resulting from a leaky gut, dysbiosis, and digestive enzyme deficiencies. Food sensitivity symptoms can vary widely from one individual to the next, depending on the type and severity of sensitivity. Common symptoms include gastrointestinal discomfort, bloating, stomach pain, excess gas, diarrhea, vomiting, nausea, acid reflux/heartburn, headaches, skin flushing, irritability or anxiety, and fatigue. These symptoms may intensify with increased consumption of the offending food and can last for several hours, or even days, after ingestion.

To manage and prevent these symptoms, you may need to avoid certain foods that cause your body's reaction. The best way to diagnose a food sensitivity or an intolerance is to work with a functional medicine provider and a dietitian or nutritionist to eliminate problem foods from your diet and then slowly reintroduce them one at a time, so you can identify the culprit. This is called a "restriction–reintroduction" diet (see next section). In addition, or alternatively, food sensitivity blood tests (such as the Cyrex assay) can be very helpful to expedite the process of identifying a much wider range of food sensitivities (especially those that may not manifest with obvious symptoms).

Some of the more common examples of food intolerances include:

- Lactose intolerance, which occurs when the lactase enzyme may be deficient and bowel symptoms occur after consuming lactose-containing foods and drinks.

- FODMAP food intolerance

- Irritable bowel syndrome (IBS), which is a common disorder that affects the digestive system. Though the exact cause of IBS is unknown, it is believed to be linked to several factors, including food sensitivities. In fact, many people with IBS find that their symptoms worsen after consuming certain foods and beverages. Common triggers include wheat, dairy products, and carbonated drinks.

- Sensitivity to food additives, such as the sulfites used to preserve dried fruits, canned goods, and wine, can trigger asthma attacks in people who are sensitive to these.

- High-histamine foods, especially those that are aged and fermented, and those that trigger histamine release (such as spinach, tomatoes, and avocados). Wine can also cause histamine release in sensitive individuals.

- Gluten intolerance (and its more severe allergic state, celiac disease), stems from consuming the gluten protein found in wheat and other grains. This protein interacts with the gut mucosa, leading to a local and possibly a systemic inflammatory and immune response (in those with celiac disease) in sensitive individuals. Symptoms often include gastrointestinal issues, as well as those unrelated to the digestive system, such as joint pain and headaches.

## Restriction–Reintroduction Diet

If you think you might have a food sensitivity, a restriction–reintroduction diet can be a helpful way to identify which foods and drinks may be causing reactions. I typically start by restricting the five most common triggers of food sensitivities for 30 days (or at least 21 days). These are gluten, dairy, soy, nuts, and eggs. Once you've eliminated these potential culprits from your diet, you can slowly reintroduce them, one at a time, monitoring your body for any signs of sensitivity. Paying close attention to how you feel after eating or drinking each item will help you narrow down which items, if any, cause sensitivity reactions. If you have any reaction to any of the foods, then you should stop eating that food.

Reintroduce foods using a 3-day cycle:

**Day 1:** Reintroduce one food, eating at least two servings of it at different times of the day. For instance, you could reintroduce eggs by having two cooked eggs at breakfast and two hard boiled eggs at lunch, perhaps in a salad. Or, when reintroducing nuts, sprinkle some on a lunchtime salad and either in another salad with dinner or in a dessert.

**Days 2 & 3:** Stop eating the new food. For example, if you reintroduced eggs on day 1, have no eggs on days 2 and 3.

**Day 4 and beyond:** What happens after day 4 will depend on how things went on days 2 and 3. If you feel good, with no effects, you'll reintroduce the next food, e.g., dairy, for one day, repeating the three day cycle. If, instead you experienced a reaction when reintroducing the previous food, wait until the symptoms totally dissipate before reintroducing another food (and continue to avoid the food that generated symptoms).

While this process takes some time and effort, it can be well worth it to finally get to the bottom of your food sensitivities.

Some people find out that they are sensitive to one or more of these five foods, and the symptoms were something their body had gotten used to over the years and, so, went unnoticed. It is similar to someone who has never worn glasses being given their first prescription.

Follow the restriction–reintroduction diet steps below. They are designed to guide anyone interested in trying this simple, effective method.

**Step 1.** Complete my Food Sensitivity Questionnaire (see page 136) and save it.

**Step 2.** Avoid all gluten, dairy, soy, nuts, and eggs ideally for 60 days, but at least 21 days.

**Step 3.** After 60 days (or however many days, but at least 21, during which you eliminated intake), retake the Food Sensitivity Questionnaire. Again, save a copy.

**Step 4.** Reintroduce your favorite food, follow the instructions on the Symptom Tracker Worksheet (see page 137) and retake the Food Sensitivity Questionnaire (optional) after four days.

**Step 5.** After 60 days, retake the Food Sensitivity Questionnaire.

**Step 6.** Repeat steps 4–6 until all five foods have been reintroduced or suspended.

The Food Sensitivity Questionnaire helps you to identify if you are sensitive to any specific foods. Again, a food *sensitivity* is different from a food *allergy*, which happens when your immune system overreacts to a harmless food protein. A food sensitivity or intolerance produces a more minor immune and inflammatory response. These can still lead to systemic and bowel symptoms, including malabsorption, which is a limited ability to absorb nutrients, minerals, and vitamins.

A true food allergy, also known as a type I hypersensitivity reaction, involves your immune system and can be life-threatening. The most common signs of a food allergy are hives, swelling in the lips or face, difficulty breathing or swallowing, and vomiting or diarrhea. Unlike with a food sensitivity, you must completely avoid foods that cause an allergic reaction to prevent a serious reaction. To diagnose a food allergy, your doctor may conduct skin or blood tests. The best way to manage a food allergy is to avoid the trigger foods completely, and carry appropriate medication (such as an EpiPen) in case of accidental exposure.

## Low-FODMAP Diet Can Improve GI Symptoms and Inflammation

Data from multiple studies have reported success in reducing these symptoms in 75% of individuals with irritable bowel syndrome using a low-FODMAP diet.

I highly recommend following a low-FODMAP diet as described in the 3-Step FODMAP Diet Guide, from Monash University (*www.monashfodmap.com/3_step_fodmap_diet*). They also have a great app, the Monash University FODMAP Diet, that you can purchase from the App Store, Google Play, or Amazon.

The aims of the diet are to:

- Learn which foods and FODMAPs you tolerate versus which trigger your symptoms, as this will help you to follow a less restrictive, more nutritionally balanced diet long term, one that only restricts the foods that trigger your symptoms.

- Assess whether your symptoms are caused by a sensitivity to FODMAPs. Not everyone with these symptoms improves on a low-FODMAP diet.

## Should You Take Probiotics, and Are There Risks?

Many of the same microbes found in our gut are also found in fermented foods, such as yogurt, kefir, kimchi, sauerkraut, miso, and healthy, unprocessed cheeses. While eating these foods has been shown to improve the health of the gut microbiome—that is, unless you have intestinal sensitivities or allergies to these foods—studies have been inconclusive about whether probiotic supplements actually improve health outcomes for everyone. You can eat them or drink them, but they won't necessarily stay and colonize the gut. Many questions remain unanswered:

- How is a specific microbiome established in an individual?
- How does our microbiome change over time?
- How does the human body and microbe community interact?
- How does a particular combination of microbes affect nutrition?
- How do changes in diet affect the microbiome?
- How does the microbiome affect immunity and contribute to disease?
- How do the microbes in our bodies affect how we respond to various drugs?
- How can a microbiome be altered to improve health?
- Which microbes are helpful, and which are not?
- How much or how often should someone consume a probiotic?

One thing we do know is that when your gut microbiome is compromised, studies have found that chemotherapy and immunotherapy may not work as well.[12] Additionally,

---

12  National Institutes of Health, "Gut microorganisms may determine cancer treatment outcome," 21 Nov. 2013, https://medicalxpress.com/news/2013-11-gut-microorganisms-cancer-treatment-outcome.html.

as noted above, there are numerous health conditions and symptoms that are associated with dysbiosis.

These findings have encouraged millions of individuals to take supplemental probiotics to try to improve their health and quality of life.

While there are certainly studies reporting numerous purported health benefits of supplemental probiotics, it's very important to note that there are also some data that have shown that these supplements may have harmful effects. For example:

- Individuals given probiotics after a course of antibiotics demonstrated a slower recovery of their normal gut microbiome than those given a placebo[13]

- Probiotic use can result in a significant accumulation of bacteria in the small intestine that can result in disorienting brain fogginess, rapid and significant belly bloating and discomfort[14]

- Probiotics given to children in an intensive care unit developed lactobacillus bacteremia[15]

- In a few cases, mainly involving individuals who were severely ill or immunocompromised, the use of probiotics has been linked to bacteremia or fungemia[16]

- Fecal transplantation of probiotic organisms (a medical approach for delivering probiotics directly into the

---

13  Jotham Suez et al., "Post-Antibiotic Gut Mucosal Microbiome Reconstitution Is Impaired by Probiotics and Improved by Autologous FMT," *Cell*, Vol. 174, Issue 6, pp. 1406–23, 6 Sept. 2018, www.cell.com/cell/fulltext/S0092-8674(18)31108-5.

14  "Probiotic use is a link between brain fogginess, severe bloating," Medical College of Georgia at Augusta University, *Science Daily*, 6 Aug. 2018, www.sciencedaily.com/releases/2018/08/180806095213.htm.

15  Idan Yelin et al., "Genomic and epidemiological evidence of bacterial transmission from probiotic capsule to blood in ICU patients," *Nature Medicine*, Vol. 25, pp. 1728–32, 7 Nov. 2019, www.nature.com/articles/s41591-019-0626-9.

16  Tina Didari et al., "A systematic review of the safety of probiotics," Expert Opinion on Drug Safety, 13:2, pp. 227–39, 3 Jan. 2014, www.ncbi.nlm.nih.gov/pubmed/24405164?dopt=Abstract.

intestines) led to an infection and subsequent death of a patient[17]

- Patients with metastatic melanoma who were taking probiotics while they were on a common immunotherapy drug were 70% less likely to respond to the immunotherapy[18]

- Certain mice in a preclinical study that were given a probiotic developed changes in the characteristics of the bacteria which caused intestinal wall damage.[19]

These studies raise questions on the generalizability of the safety of supplementing with probiotics. While there are no hard and fast rules on contraindications for taking probiotics, these are some of the more common recommendations for who should be more cautious with their use:

- Patients with a central venous catheter

- Patients who are critically ill

- Patients with severely suppressed immune systems, including people with low white-blood-cell counts (neutropenia) as a result of cancer treatment

- Individuals with sensitivities or allergies to specific probiotics

- Individuals taking certain medications for which there are drug–probiotic interactions

- Patients taking immunotherapy drugs

My recommendation is to check with your cancer care team before taking a probiotic supplement and ask them whether

---

17  Kate Sheridan, "Massachusetts General Hospital oversaw trial that led to the first death from a fecal transplant, a new paper shows," *STAT*, 30 Oct. 2019, www.statnews.com/2019/10/30/details-first-death-fecal-transplant.

18  Meghana Keshavan, "Probiotics are touted as good for the gut. They may be trouble for the immune system," *STAT*, 2 Apr. 2019, www.statnews.com/2019/04/02/probiotics-are-touted-as-good-for-the-gut-they-may-be-trouble-for-the-immune-system.

19  Ana Sandoiu, "Could probiotics evolve in the gut and cause harm?" *Medical News Today*, 29 Mar. 2019, www.medicalnewstoday.com/articles/324834.php#4.

you can safely eat foods containing live bacteria. If they advise against this, do what you can to consume prebiotics— vegetables, fruits, whole grains, beans, etc.—to support the health of the microbes that live in your gut.

## Customized Probiotics

It is important to recognize is that there is no one-size-fits-all probiotic supplement or food. If you are like me and believe the studies that suggest that taking a probiotic improves gut and systemic health in those with dysbiosis, I recommend that you start by undergoing a stool microbiome test (such as the GI MAP test) to assess for dysbiosis. If my patients have dysbiosis, I suggest they consider taking measures to specifically address their mix of organisms:

- Those with high or low levels (outside the reference ranges) of microbes should increase their intake of prebiotics and address the points noted in the section on Gut Health starting on page 53
- Those who have gastrointestinal symptoms (such as bloating, cramping, diarrhea) and high levels of pathogenic ("bad") microbes might need to be treated with an antimicrobial dietary supplement and/or medication (such as antibiotics, anti-parasitics, and antifungals)
- Those with low levels of specific microbes can be addressed with targeted supplementation

Targeted probiotic supplementation should be based on lab testing, as there is no other way to know which organisms are deficient. An important added complexity is that, over time (days to years), one's microbiome is constantly changing, therefore you may need to continue to test for these changes and adjust the probiotic supplementation as needed.

Sun Genomics (*flore.com*) has developed a commercial probiotic, FLORÉ Precision Probiotics, based on the results of a stool DNA test. Customers submit a stool sample to the Sun Genomics lab, which ships back a customized three-month supply of probiotics to help address the customers' dysbiosis. Every few months, stool testing is repeated and modifications to the probiotic supplements are made. In my experience working with patients, this is the best supplemental probiotic approach currently available to help address gut dysbiosis.

## Polyphenols Feed Your Microbiome

The plants you consume are not only great for their prebiotic benefits but also contain important compounds called polyphenols. Dietary polyphenols are present in fruits and vegetables, certain cereals (barley, rye, oats, wheat and wheat bran, couscous, cocoa, flaxseed), tea, coffee, and red wine, among others.

Studies have illustrated their antioxidant, anti-inflammatory, anti-diabetic, anti-cancer, neuroprotective, and fat-loss properties. The benefit of their poor absorption is that polyphenols are retained in the intestine longer, where they enhance the growth, balance, and diversity of your gut microbiome.[20]

---

20  César G. Fraga et al., "The effects of polyphenols and other bioactives on human health," *Food & Function*, 12 Feb 2019, 10, pp. 514–528, https://pubs.rsc.org/en/content/articlehtml/2019/fo/c8fo01997e.

# A Functional Medicine Approach to Optimize Gut Health

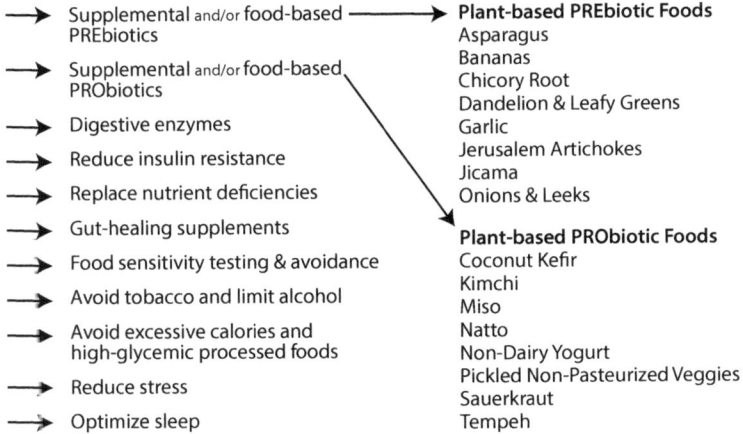

→ Supplemental and/or food-based
  PREbiotics

→ Supplemental and/or food-based
  PRObiotics

→ Digestive enzymes

→ Reduce insulin resistance

→ Replace nutrient deficiencies

→ Gut-healing supplements

→ Food sensitivity testing & avoidance

→ Avoid tobacco and limit alcohol

→ Avoid excessive calories and
  high-glycemic processed foods

→ Reduce stress

→ Optimize sleep

→ **Plant-based PREbiotic Foods**
Asparagus
Bananas
Chicory Root
Dandelion & Leafy Greens
Garlic
Jerusalem Artichokes
Jicama
Onions & Leeks

**Plant-based PRObiotic Foods**
Coconut Kefir
Kimchi
Miso
Natto
Non-Dairy Yogurt
Pickled Non-Pasteurized Veggies
Sauerkraut
Tempeh

# Toxins

It is important to consider the role that toxins play in our overall health and well-being. Our bodies are literally full of toxins that we accumulate from exposures in our diet, environment, lifestyle, and those produced naturally as byproducts within our tissues. These can have a wide range of negative health impacts, which is why it's so important to assess and address these when optimizing your health.

Some common types of toxins that can have significant effects on our health include pesticides, heavy metals, mold toxins, and industrial chemicals. Because there are so many different types of toxins out there in the world today—both natural and manmade—it's essential to be aware of how these can affect your health, and to take steps to minimize your exposures.

## Smoking Tobacco

Smoking tobacco has been linked to a wide range of chronic health conditions, including cardiovascular disease, chronic obstructive pulmonary disease, cancer, atherosclerosis, asthma, ulcers, periodontal disease, and others. Tobacco exposes you to a host of toxins: cadmium, carbon monoxide, acetone, formaldehyde, ammonia, arsenic, hydrogen cyanide, methane, butane, and even the pesticide DDT, to name just a few.

Cancer patients who continue to smoke while undergoing treatment have been shown to experience significantly worse outcomes. Quitting smoking is one of the best things you can do for your health, and there are a variety of resources available to help you quit. Talk to your doctor about what quitting-smoking methods may be right for you.

## Alcohol

Alcohol consumption is a known risk factor for the development of multiple cancers. This is believed to be due to the toxic byproduct of alcohol breakdown, acetaldehyde, which can cause DNA damage. Emerging evidence[21] suggests that even moderate drinking (three or more drinks per week) may increase the risk for cancers of the mouth, throat, esophagus, liver, breast and bowel.

If you are concerned about your cancer risk, it is important to talk to your doctor about your drinking habits and whether or not they may be putting you at increased risk.

## Pesticides

Pesticides in our produce can also damage our DNA, gut, brain and metabolic health. These compounds are ubiquitous in non-organic fruits and vegetables, which is why we need to be thoughtful in our selection of our produce. The nonprofit Environmental Working Group (EWG) annually releases their list of the "dirty dozen" and "clean 15" produce items (*www.ewg.org/foodnews*). Their annual pesticide list ranks pesticide-laden produce numerically, from the most to least toxic produce items in the market.

While there is a lot of debate in the scientific community about whether non-organic fruits and vegetables—those

---

21 "Update of Canada's Low-Risk Alcohol Drinking Guidelines: Final Report for Public Consultation," Canadian Centre on Substance Use and Addiction, August 2022, https://www.ccsa.ca/sites/default/files/2022-08/CCSA-LRDG-Update-of-Canada%27s-LRDG-Final-report-for-public-consultation-en.pdf.

exposed to pesticides and other farming chemicals—cause serious health problems, I recommend that, until we know more conclusively of the potential risks, when buying produce that is on the EWG "dirty dozen" list (the most chemically laden produce) to choose the organic versions whenever possible. You can save your money on those produce items listed on the "clean 15" (least chemically laden) list by buying the non-organic versions if you so choose.

## Fish

When choosing fish, there are potential concerns regarding toxins and environmental sustainability. I recommend using the EWG Consumer Guide to Seafood (*www.ewg. org/consumer-guides/ewgs-consumer-guide-seafood*) when choosing less toxic fish, and the Monterey Bay Aquarium Seafood Watch Guides (*www.seafoodwatch.org/seafood-recommendations/consumer-guides*) to help select the most environmentally sustainable options.

## Toxic Food Ingredients

Toxic food ingredients are also a concern. The EWG Healthy Living app (*www.ewg.org/apps*) can help you select foods that are the least toxic. The app rates foods from 1 to 10, with 1 being the cleanest and 10 being the most toxic on their scale. You can also use the app to identify alternative food items in the same category that are less toxic.

The app is a great resource for helping you make healthier choices when it comes to the food you eat. By avoiding foods that are high on the EWG scale, you can help reduce your exposure to harmful chemicals and toxins. So, next time you're at the store, be sure to check the app before you buy anything.

## Personal Care Product Toxins

Toxins in personal care products are also very commonplace. The Campaign for Safe Cosmetics (*www.safecosmetics.org*) and the Environmental Working Group have resources that can help you select the least toxic personal care products. The EWG's Skin Deep app (*www.ewg.org/skindeep*) and their Guide to Sunscreens (*www.ewg.org/sunscreen*) can help you identify specific products, which it ranks from best to worst based on ingredient concerns. The Campaign for Safe Cosmetics shares information on top products and contaminants to avoid, and steps you can take to reduce toxic exposures that will protect your health and the health of your family.

## Cleaning Product Toxins

As with cosmetics, many household cleaning products contain toxic chemicals. I recommend using the EWG Guide to Healthy Cleaning (*www.ewg.org/guides/cleaners*) to help you select the least toxic household cleaning products.

## Toxins in Tap Water

Potentially unsafe levels of lead, arsenic, the "forever chemicals" known as PFAS, and many other substances are often found in drinking water. EWG's Tap Water Database (*www.ewg.org/tapwater*) shows how polluted drinking water can be. The database comprises annual test reports from 2014 to 2019, produced by almost 50,000 U.S. water utilities in all 50 states and the District of Columbia. It reveals that when some Americans drink a glass of tap water, they're also potentially getting a dose of industrial or agricultural contaminants linked to cancer, brain and nervous system damage, fertility problems, hormone disruption, and other health problems.

If your utility is listed as having unsafe levels of contaminants, you can take steps to protect yourself and your family by using a home water filter or avoiding drinking tap water altogether. Visit EWG's Tap Water Database today to see how your drinking water stacks up. You can also use the EWGs Water Filter Guide (*www.ewg.org/tapwater/water-filter-guide.php*) to help you choose the right filter for your water and budget.

## Assessing and Addressing Your Toxic Burden

It's estimated that, on average, we ingest 700–2,000 ppm (parts per million) of potentially toxic chemicals daily. To put this in perspective, there is no known safe level of exposure to any toxin. In fact, according to the EPA, the Environmental Protection Agency, even brief exposures to small amounts of toxins can be unsafe. Pharmaceuticals, pesticides, packaged foods, household products, and environmental pollution all contribute to our exposure. Many of these chemicals have been associated with increased risks of developing chronic illnesses, like cancer, heart disease, chronic fatigue syndrome, chemical sensitivity, ADHD, autoimmune disorders, Parkinson's disease, and Alzheimer's disease.

There are a variety of ways to test for chemicals that have accumulated in your body over time. The three main tests I recommend for assessing one's toxic load are the NutrEval lab test and Mosaic Diagnostics GPL-TOX and MycoTOX profile tests.

# Mold Testing
## (MOSAIC, Myco-TOX Profile Sample Report)

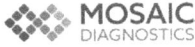

**MOSAIC DIAGNOSTICS**  **MycoTOX PROFILE**

| Requisition #: | 9900001 | Practitioner | NO PHYSICIAN |
| Patient Name: | Report Sample | Date of Collection: | Dec 1, 2022 |
| Date of Birth: | Apr 10, 2005 | Time of Collection: | Not Given |
| Gender: | M | Print Date: | Mar 21, 2023 |
| | | Report Date: | December 01, 2021 |

## Mycotox Profile

Creatinine Value: 100.00 mg/dl

| Metabolite | Results (ng/g creatinine) | Normal Range * | Abnormal Range |
|---|---|---|---|
| **Aspergillus** | | | |
| Aflatoxin-M1 | 23.00 | < 0.5 | ▲ 0.5 |
| Ochratoxin A | 54.00 | < 7.5 | ▲ 7.5 |
| Gliotoxin | 205.00 | < 200 | ▲ 200 |
| **Penicillium** | | | |
| Sterigmatocystin | 64.00 | < 0.4 | ▲ 0.4 |

*\* The normal range was calculated using the median + 2 times the standard deviation*

Testing performed by The Great Plains Laboratory, LLC., Overland Park, Kansas. The Great Plains Laboratory has developed and determined the performance characteristics of this test. The test has not been evaluated by the U.S. Food and Drug Administration. The FDA does not currently regulate such testing.

Page 1 of 9

Angela Purvis, PhD, NRCC | 9221 Quivira Road, Overland Park, KS 66215 | (913) 341-8949 | Fax: (913) 341-6207 | MosaicDX.com

# Toxin Testing
## (MOSAIC, GPL-TOX Profile Sample Report)

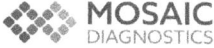

**MOSAIC** DIAGNOSTICS                                    **GPL-TOX** PROFILE

| | | | | | | |
|---|---|---|---|---|---|---|
| Requisition #: | 9900001 | | | Practitioner: | NO PHYSICIAN | |
| Patient Name: | Report Sample | | | Date of Collection: | 12/01/2022 | |
| Date Of Birth: | 04/10/2005 | Patient Age: | 17 | Time of Collection: | Not Given | |
| Sex: | M | | | Print Date: | 3/21/2023 | |
| | | | | Report Date: | 12/01/2021 | |

## Toxic Compounds

| Metabolite | Result µg/g creatinine | Percentile |
|---|---|---|

**1) 2-Hydroxyisobutyric Acid (2HIB)** — 6,321

| LLOQ | | 75th | 95th |
|---|---|---|---|
| 200 | | 7,493 | 11,908 |

*Parent: MTBE/ETBE*
MTBE and ETBE are gasoline additives used to improve octane ratings. Exposure to these compounds is most likely due to groundwater contamination, inhalation or skin exposure to gasoline or its vapors, and exhaust fumes. MTBE has been demonstrated to cause hepatic, kidney, and central nervous system toxicity, peripheral neurotoxicity, and cancer in animals. Very high values have been reported in genetic disorders. Because the metabolites of these compounds are the same, ETBE may be similarly toxic.

**2) Monoethylphthalate (MEP)** — 33

| LLOQ | 75th | | 95th |
|---|---|---|---|
| 5.0 | 73 | | 374 |

*Parent: Diethylphthalates*
Phthalates may be the most widespread group of toxins in our environment, commonly found in many bath and beauty products, cosmetics, perfumes, oral pharmaceuticals, insect repellants, adhesives, inks, and varnishes. Phthalates have been implicated in reproductive damage, depressed leukocyte function, and cancer. Phthalates have also been found to impede blood coagulation, lower testosterone, and alter sexual development in children. Low levels of phthalates can feminize the male brain of the fetus, while high levels can hyper-masculinize the developing male brain.

**3) 2-3-4 Methylhippuric Acid (2,3,4 MHA)** — 72

| LLOQ | 75th | | 95th |
|---|---|---|---|
| 10 | 603 | | 1,623 |

*Parent: Xylene*
Xylenes (dimethylbenzenes) are found not only in common products such as paints, lacquers, pesticides, cleaning fluids, fuel and exhaust fumes, but also in perfumes and insect repellants. Xylenes are oxidized in the liver and bound to glycine before eliminated in urine. High exposures to xylene create an increase in oxidative stress, causing symptoms such as nausea, vomiting, dizziness, central nervous system depression, and death. Occupational exposure is often found in pathology laboratories where xylene is used for tissue processing.

*LLOQ - Lower Limit of Quantitation                                    **N.D. - Not Detected

Testing performed by The Great Plains Laboratory, LLC., Overland Park, Kansas. The Great Plains Laboratory has developed and determined the performance characteristics of this test. This test has not been evaluated by the U.S. FDA; the FDA does not currently regulate such testing

Page 1 of 16

Angela Purvis, PhD, NRCC | 9221 Quivira Road, Overland Park, KS 66215 | (913) 341-8949 | Fax: (913) 341-6207 | MosaicDX.com

## Toxin Metal Testing
### (Genova Diagnostics, NutrEval Sample Report)

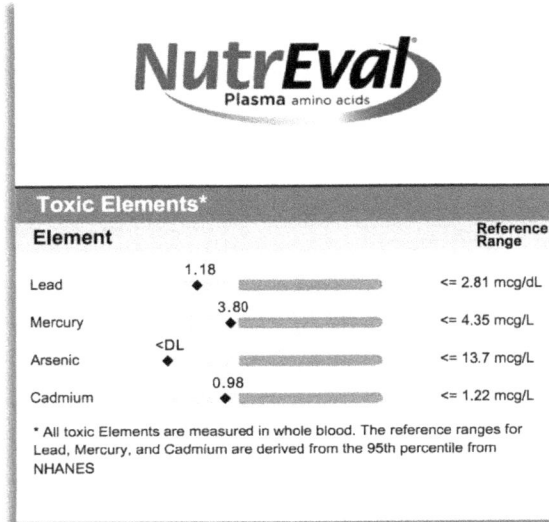

## NutrEval

The Genova NutrEval test predominantly looks at one's nutrient status; however, it also reports toxic metal levels and chemical metabolites within the body that are produced after toxic exposure. Importantly, many of the nutrients often found to be deficient are the very ones involved in detoxification pathways. Addressing these deficiencies can help improve one's natural detoxification processes and lower their toxic body burden. Additionally, adding certain supplements or other detoxification methods can also be used.

# Liver Detoxification Pathways:
### Phase 1 and Phase 2

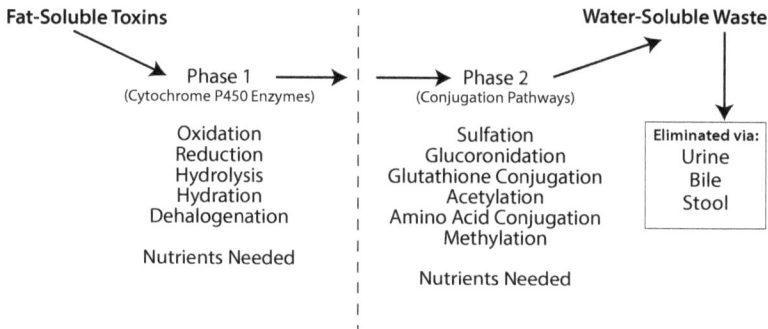

**Fat-Soluble Toxins**

**Water-Soluble Waste**

Phase 1
(Cytochrome P450 Enzymes)

Phase 2
(Conjugation Pathways)

Oxidation
Reduction
Hydrolysis
Hydration
Dehalogenation

Sulfation
Glucoronidation
Glutathione Conjugation
Acetylation
Amino Acid Conjugation
Methylation

Eliminated via:
Urine
Bile
Stool

Nutrients Needed

Nutrients Needed

## GPL-TOX

The Mosaic Diagnostics GPL-TOX test can help you identify your exposure to a variety of toxic chemicals, allowing you to take steps to reduce your risk of chronic disease. This profile screens for 173 different toxic chemicals, including organophosphate pesticides, phthalates, benzene, xylene, vinyl chloride, pyrethroid insecticides, acrylamide, perchlorate, diphenyl phosphate, ethylene oxide, acrylonitrile, and more. By knowing which toxins you are exposed to, you can make beneficial lifestyle changes to reduce your exposure and protect your health.

## Mycotoxins

Mycotoxins are among the most prevalent toxins in our environment. These chemical compounds are produced by fungal organisms, which can grow everywhere, from buildings and vehicles to foodstuffs. Fungi can grow on almost any surface, especially if the environment is warm and wet. Inner wall materials of buildings, such as wallpaper, fiberglass insulation, ceiling tiles, and gypsum support, are all conducive surfaces for fungi to colonize. These fungi release mycotoxins into the environment that can cause asthma, sinusitis, memory and cognitive impairment, chronic fatigue, skin rashes, depression, ADHD, anxiety, and systemic inflammation. The link between mycotoxin exposures and cancer risk has been established in studies with the consumption of aflatoxin-contaminated foods and primary liver cancer in humans. While the link with other mycotoxins and cancer types has mainly been established in experimental studies, further research is necessary to support these associations in human epidemiological studies.[22]

## MycoTOX

The Mosaic Diagnostics MycoTOX Profile is one of the most comprehensive mycotoxin tests available, screening for eleven different mycotoxins from 40 species of mold in a single urine sample. This allows us to identify mycotoxin exposures and make recommendations for detoxification treatments that have been effective.

## Fungus/Mold Mitigation

Testing for molds and fungi in places where one spends a significant amount of time (such as their home or office) may be necessary to try to identify the potential source of one's exposure. Mold inspection specialists (such as *yesweinspect. com*) and mitigation/removal contractors (such as *homecleanse. com*) are often needed in these circumstances. Working with a mold sickness specialist (such as Jill Crista, N.D., *drcrista.com*, or Neil Nathan, M.D., *neilnathanmd.com*) and/or an infectious disease doctor to help manage mold illnesses and symptoms

22   Liesel Claeys et al., "Mycotoxin exposure and human cancer risk: A systematic review of epidemiological studies," Comprehensive Reviews in Food Science and Food Safety, Vol. 19, Issue 4, pp. 1449–64, 20 May 2020, doi. org/10.1111/1541-4337.12567.

is recommended for anyone who has lab testing confirmation of high levels of mold exposure or is symptomatic.

## Methylation Activity and the DUTCH Plus Test

I recommend testing for one's methylation activity, as methylation is one of the most important methods the body employs to detoxify chemicals. Methylation is also one of the main methods in which the body activates and deactivates genes, and converts hormones such as estrogen into downstream metabolites. Some of these estrogen metabolites are associated with estrogen receptor stimulation. Knowing that one has an excess of these undesirable stimulating estrogen metabolites (such as 4-OH and 16-OH estrogen) can help us to make recommendations to reverse this process and promote greater production of more desirable, less stimulating metabolites, such as 2-OH estrogen. DIM, or diindolylmethane, is one such supplement that promotes 2-OH estrogen production and is also found in cruciferous vegetables like broccoli, Brussels sprouts, cabbage, and kale, while vitamin A, vitamin C, vitamin E, glutathione, N-acetyl-cysteine, and selenomethionine mitigate the effects of quinones, which are the dangerous 4-OH estrogen metabolites.

The DUTCH Plus is my favorite test to assess methylation activity and estrogen metabolites. As mentioned earlier, this test also assesses your overall daily levels of free cortisol, cortisol metabolites, sex hormones and their metabolites, oxidative stress, and melatonin.

## Minimizing Our Toxic Burden

Minimizing our toxic burden requires a multipronged approach. One of the first steps is to assess your baseline toxic burden with the recommended lab tests mentioned above. This is not required for most, but it will help you track your progress over time and give you an idea of how well your interventions are working. You'll want to revisit these labs over time as well, since we're constantly exposed to new toxins (e.g., BPA in plastic; mercury in fish) and concentrations change based on your exposure and how much is eliminated from your system through detoxification pathways.

Once you've assessed your toxic burden and potential contributing risk factors (such as nutrient deficiencies, systemic inflammation, impaired gut health, low methylation activity, etc.), the next steps are lifestyle related and include minimizing toxic exposure, reducing stress, encouraging regular exercise, ensuring regular bowel movements, consuming adequate amounts of fiber and prebiotic foods, sweating, ensuring adequate hydration, and sleep. The figure below lists the steps to take to reduce the burden of toxins on your body.

## A Functional Medicine Approach to Reducing Toxic Body Burden

Toxins

Dark Gray boxes: Assess metal toxins with the NutrEval test, and non-metal & mold toxins with the Mosaic Diagnostics tests.

| NutrEval | Mosaic Diagnostics |
|---|---|

Medium Gray boxes: Address potential contributing factors to toxic body burden

| Minimize Toxic Exposure | |
|---|---|
| >/= One Bowel Movement per day | |
| Toxin-Clearing Supplements | Fiber, Prebiotics |

| Exercise | Sleep | Hydration | Sauna |
|---|---|---|---|

Light Gray boxes: Consider additional functional medicine testing for variables that can influence toxic body burden

| Systemic Inflammation | Nutrients |
|---|---|
| Low 2-OH Estrogen | Low Methylation |
| Dysbiosis, Leaky Gut, Gut Inflammation, Food Sensitivities | |

# Functional Drug Sensitivity/ Chemosensitivity Testing

When choosing cancer drugs for our patients, we rely on guidelines such as those from NCCN, National Comprehensive Cancer Network. However, one major problem with following a consensus-based guideline is that it can't answer the million-dollar question: *Will this person's cancer die when we use X, Y, or Z drug(s)?* What I mean by this is: How do we know that this particular person's cancer will respond to any specific drug, or combination of drugs, recommended by the guidelines? The answer is that we don't know, not until we treat them and see what happens.

For some cancers (lymphomas, leukemias, testicular cancers), we have seen remarkable effectiveness with guidelines-based drug therapies. Unfortunately, not all cancers (i.e., gastric, pancreatic, lung, melanoma, glioblastoma multiforme, ovarian) are as exquisitely sensitive to the standard drug regimens recommended by the consensus guidelines.

Most medical oncologists have limited their use of precision medicine testing to "next generation sequencing" (NGS) genetic assays (such as FoundationOne CDX, Foundation Medicine) to detect genomic abnormalities in certain cancers, and depending on the results of these assays, they may prescribe a drug targeting the detected abnormality. These types of assays don't tell us whether the drug will actually kill your cancer; however, they do give us a hint that it might work. Unfortunately, the effectiveness of this approach has not been dramatic when used against many cancers, with response rates of two to six months, on average. However, in some cancer types with identified genomic targets (such as ALK, EGFR, BRCA), the responses can be much greater.

With the growing availability of precision cancer therapies, patients now have more options when it comes to treating their cancer. These treatments are designed specifically for each individual patient, taking into account the unique characteristics of their tumor and other factors that may impact how well a drug will work.

One such precision medicine test that is gaining popularity (although still not commonly used) among oncologists is a functional drug sensitivity (or chemosensitivity) assay. This test involves removing a small, fresh piece of tumor tissue (either tissue biopsy, malignant pleural fluid, or malignant ascites fluid) from a patient's body using a minimally invasive procedure, creating 3-D tumor microspheroids (microscopic clusters of cells), which contain tumor cells and tumor stromal cells (non-cancerous cells that comprise the scaffolding and blood supply in your tumor). In the lab, these microspheroids are methodically analyzed, after subjecting them individually to various cancer drugs, to determine which drugs or combination of drugs caused the greatest amount of microspheroid cell death. The results of this chemosensitivity test enables your oncologist to predict which of the tested drugs has the greatest chance of being effective against your cancer.

The test results can take anywhere from a few days up to several months to see which drug, or drugs, actually work. Labs have been developing a variety of personalized assays using microspheroids, such as that described above, and in mouse (*in vivo*) studies to see how sensitive a patient's cancer is to the drugs tested. Keep in mind that these are not perfect assays, as they cannot account for innumerable physiological variables in an individual. However, studies comparing outcomes from patients who received personalized drug regimens using modern chemosensitivity tests have found significantly improved cancer outcomes (including better cancer response rates and better survival) compared with those who were not treated with the benefit of these tests. The development, validation, and clinical implementation of these assays is one of the most exciting areas in oncology today.

Numerous top academic cancer centers (such as Harvard, Weill Cornell Medicine, Sunnybrook Research Institute, and many others) are developing their own versions of these state-of-the-art drug sensitivity assays, but most are still in the research and development stage.

The drug sensitivity assay I recommend most frequently among those currently available is the Nagourney Cancer Institute's EVA-PCD Functional Profile, also known as the Ex-Vivo Analysis of Programmed Death (*www.nagourneycancerinstitute.com*).

The details will vary depending on the assay but, in general, to get these tests done, you will need:
- to take about two to four weeks off from most cancer drug therapies.
- depending on the cancer type, have your doctors collect either blood if you have leukemia, bone marrow if you have leukemia or myeloma, tumor tissue if solid tumors are present, or malignant effusions (pleural fluid or ascites fluid.) *NOTE: Obtaining a sample of your tumor to submit for testing is not a risk-free procedure. Discuss with your oncologist whether the potential risks outweigh the potential benefits in your situation.*
- Submit the sample to the lab. This can be done through same-day or overnight delivery services, such as FedEx, in special packaging.

- Wait for the results. Depending on the test, this may take only one to two weeks to get your results. These will be sent directly to your oncologist.
- Talk with your oncologist about which regimen makes the most sense for you, based on your assay results and other factors.

## First-Generation Clonogenic Chemo-Sensitivity Assays

The first-generation (and much less accurate) chemosensitivity assays used colonies of clonogenic (cloned) cancer cells or cancer stem cells, instead of fresh, whole-tissue biopsy specimens (which include tumor cells and microenvironment cells), and subjected them to chemotherapy drugs. Unfortunately, there were many flaws in this approach:

- Clonogenic cells acquire mutations that make them behave very differently to the tumor cells in your body.
- Since the patient's tumor microenvironment cells were not incorporated into these first-generation assays, real-world tumor response was not accurate. We now know that these tumor microenvironment and immune cells interact with tumor cells and can either enhance or reduce the efficacy of various drug therapies.
- Circulating tumor cell (CTC) assays collect free-floating cancer cells from the blood, but these CTCs may not manifest the same behavior—i.e., cell death—in the presence of drugs as they do in whole-tissue assays. One such test is the Onconomics RGCC ("Greek Test"), which claims that it can test numerous drugs against CTCs collected from the blood.

It is not surprising that these flawed, first-generation chemosensitivity assays did a poor job of predicting the most effective drugs for the tumors treated. In 2004, ASCO reviewers concluded that these assays were not useful.[23]

---

23  Deborah Schrag et al., American Society of Clinical Oncology Technology

Unfortunately, many oncologists have not yet embraced the latest, second-generation chemosensitivity assays (i.e., the EVA-PCD assay), believing that all chemosensitivity assays are equally flawed.

The latest functional drug sensitivity (chemo-sensitivity) assays use fresh, live tumor tissue (or ascites/pleural fluid), which has led to a much more accurate prognostic response to drug therapies. In addition to the Nagourney Cancer Institute's EVA-PCD assay, others that are commercially available and worth exploring are SEngine's Paris test (*senginemedicine.com/paris-test*) and ASC Oncology test (*www.asc-oncology.com/en/home*).

These tests are not typically covered by insurance. The cost depends on the drugs tested, but is approximately $4,000; this does not include the procedure cost of the sample collection (i.e., biopsy, etc.) or the shipping.[24]

---

Assessment: Chemotherapy Sensitivity and Resistance Assays, *Journal of Clinical Oncology*, 22, no. 17, 1 Sep. 2004, pp. 3631–38. https://ascopubs.org/doi/full/10.1200/JCO.2004.05.065?role=tab.

24  For more information, visit the Nagourney Cancer Institute website at www.nagourneycancerinstitute.com or call them at 800-542-4357.

# Cancer Screening:
# Your Risk of a New Cancer

There are numerous cancer risk assessment tools that are available to you, for free. For example, *Reduce My Risk* (*risk.oncolink.org*) is one tool to help you learn about factors that affect your personal risk of many types of cancer and—most importantly—what you can do to decrease your risk.

To help increase awareness of cancer risk factors and to aid in early cancer detection, here is a link to 34 risk calculators (*www.calculators.org/health/cancer.php*) for different types of cancer.

## Everyone Should Be Offered Genetic Testing

I feel that every individual who has ever been diagnosed with cancer should be offered hereditary cancer genetic testing, because a diagnosis of cancer is a risk factor for developing future cancers. A Mayo Clinic study of nearly 3,000 patients with cancer found that one in eight patients with a solid tumor cancer have a genetic mutation that is known to be related to the development of various cancers.[25] Importantly, 50% of these individuals would not have been recommended

---

25   N. Jewel Samadder, et al., "Comparison of Universal Genetic Testing vs. Guideline-Directed Targeted Testing for Patients with Hereditary Cancer Syndrome," *JAMA Oncology*, 30 Oct. 2020, pp. 230–37, https://jamanetwork.com/journals/jamaoncology/fullarticle/2772576.

to undergo genetic testing based on the current guidelines. Furthermore, nearly one-third of these patients were found to be carrying a mutation that led to a change in their treatment.

A study of 3,607 men with a personal history of prostate cancer found that 17.2% carried a hereditary genetic mutation predisposing them to cancer.[26] Importantly, 37% of these men did not qualify for genetic testing per the recommended expert guidelines and thus would not have been offered testing.

A similar study in breast cancer patients found that basing genetic testing on established guidelines will lead to missing nearly 50% of those who carry a high risk mutation,[27] which is why the American Society of Breast Surgeons now recommends offering genetic testing for ALL breast cancer patients.[28]

Did you know that 10–15% of all cancers are due, in part, to genetic mutations inherited from our parents? This is why I recommend that even if you have no prior history of cancer, knowing if you carry a mutation that is associated with having an increased risk for developing cancer should be an option for everyone.

I recommend getting a multi-gene panel test to identify cancer-promoting genetic mutations (such as BRCA and many others) that you may have inherited from your parents. Knowing whether you carry one or more of these mutations can help inform you and your healthcare provider on:

- when to start and how frequently you should get cancer screening tests

---

26  Piper Nicolosi, et al., "Prevalence of Germline Variants in Prostate Cancer and Implications for Current Genetic Testing Guidelines," *JAMA Oncology*, 7 Feb. 2019, pp. 523–28, https://jamanetwork.com/article.aspx?doi=10.1001/jamaoncol.2018.6760.

27  Peter D. Beitsch, et al., "Underdiagnosis of Hereditary Breast Cancer: Are Genetic Testing Guidelines a Tool or an Obstacle?," *Journal of Clinical Oncology*, Vol. 37, Issue 36, 20 Feb. 2019, https://ascopubs.org/doi/full/10.1200/JCO.18.01631.

28  See www.breastsurgeons.org/docs/statements/Consensus-Guideline-on-Genetic-Testing-for-Hereditary-Breast-Cancer.pdf.

- implementing cancer risk reduction and preventive measures
- counseling your family members on their hereditary cancer risk and offering appropriate genetic testing

There are many hereditary cancer genetic tests on the market. I most commonly recommend multi-gene panels from Myriad, Invitae, Color, and Natera. You can ask your healthcare provider to order these for you, but insurance will only cover these tests if your hereditary cancer risks are high enough to meet the guidelines indications for testing. If you do not meet these insurance criteria for testing, you can still get these tests done, but it will be out of pocket. (Some cost less than $300.) Fortunately, you only need to have this test, usually performed with either a blood or cheek swab sample, done once in your lifetime.

## Cancer Screening

Since 40% of us will develop cancer in our lifetime, early cancer detection through screening is one of the most important things we can do to increase our longevity. In the vast majority of cases, the earlier we can detect a cancer, the better the outcome.

# How to Detect Cancer as Early as Possible

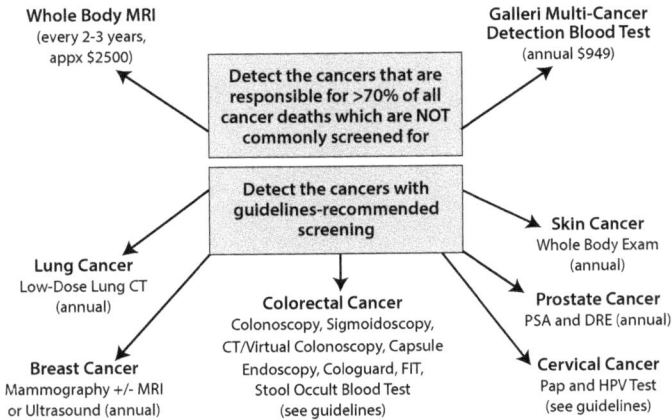

**Whole Body MRI**
(every 2-3 years,
appx $2500)

**Galleri Multi-Cancer Detection Blood Test**
(annual $949)

Detect the cancers that are responsible for >70% of all cancer deaths which are NOT commonly screened for

Detect the cancers with guidelines-recommended screening

**Skin Cancer**
Whole Body Exam
(annual)

**Lung Cancer**
Low-Dose Lung CT
(annual)

**Colorectal Cancer**
Colonoscopy, Sigmoidoscopy,
CT/Virtual Colonoscopy, Capsule
Endoscopy, Cologuard, FIT,
Stool Occult Blood Test
(see guidelines)

**Prostate Cancer**
PSA and DRE (annual)

**Breast Cancer**
Mammography +/- MRI
or Ultrasound (annual)

**Cervical Cancer**
Pap and HPV Test
(see guidelines)

**Breast Cancer Screening (female):**
- Starting at age 40 (average risk)
- Annual mammogram and breast examination

**Cervical Cancer Screening (female):**
- Starting at age 21: Pap smear every 3 years
- Age 30–65: HPV test and Pap smear every 5 years

**Colorectal Cancer Screening:**
- Start at age 45 (average risk)
- Colonoscopy every 10 years (if normal) or
- Cologuard every 3 years (if normal)

**Head & Neck (including thyroid) Cancer Screening:**
- Annual physical exam (all ages)

**Hereditary Cancer Genetic Mutation Screening:**
- Only need to test once using a multi-gene assay (all ages)

**Prostate Cancer Screening (male):**
- Start at age 40
- Annual PSA blood test + digital rectal exam (if PSA >/=2ng/mL)

**Skin Cancer Screening:**
- Annual physical exam (all ages)

**Testicular Cancer Screening (male):**
- Annual physical exam (all ages)

**Total Body Cancer Screening:**
- Annual physical exam (all ages)
- Annual Galleri blood test (No standard recommendations. Consider starting at age 50. Those with cancer risk factors can consider starting at age 40)
- Whole body MRI (No standard recommendations. Consider starting at age 50); Every 1-3 years

**Toxin Testing:**
- Annual toxic metals and chemical testing (any age)

**Lung Cancer Screening:**
Annual low-dose chest CT scan (50–80 years old and a >/=20-pack year smoking history and smoke now or have quit within the past 15-years. Those who have high-risk occupations of toxic smoke inhalation, such as firefighters with 20+ years of occupational exposure, should also consider annual low-dose chest CT screening.)

In addition to inherited genetic mutations, one of the most common risk factors for developing cancer is having had a prior history of cancer. This is why it's even more important for cancer patients and survivors to get their recommended cancer screenings. While current guidelines recommend that we screen for breast, prostate, colorectal, cervical, and lung cancers, over 70% of all cancer deaths are caused by other cancer types, ones not commonly screened for.

## Galleri Blood Test

Among the 12 cancers that are responsible for two-thirds of all cancer deaths per year in the U.S., there is a state-of-the-art blood test that can detect these with a 76% sensitivity: the Galleri test, by Grail. It can detect the presence of over 50 different cancers with one simple blood draw. The Galleri blood test is also able to identify the site of the cancer's origin in the body with an 89% accuracy. Based on a clinical study, 1% of tested individuals received a positive result ("cancer signal detected"). After further diagnostic evaluation (such as imaging studies, additional lab testing and/or biopsies), around 40% of people received a confirmed cancer diagnosis (positive predictive value). In a separate study, 0.5% of individuals without a cancer diagnosis received a positive result (false positive).

It's estimated that if the Galleri test were added to routine cancer screenings, the number of cancers detected in adults in the U.S. through screening could increase from 200,000 a year to over 600,000 a year, *a three-fold increase in cancer detection.*

Why is this test such a huge breakthrough? Because earlier detection of cancers often means better survival outcomes for our patients. Data show that the five-year cancer mortality rate for all cancers is 79% when detected late versus 11% with early detection.

The Galleri test is recommended to be done annually, *in addition* to guideline-recommended cancer screenings such as mammography, colonoscopy, PSA (prostate specific-membrane antigen), cervical cancer (Pap smear and HPV testing), and lung cancer (low-dose lung CT scan) screening.

Galleri is recommended for use in *any* adult (but never for any patient under 21) with an elevated risk of cancer, such as those 50 or older, those with a personal or family history of cancer, or *anyone* interested in early cancer detection. If a cancer signal is detected on a Galleri test, your healthcare provider will complete a diagnostic workup for further evaluation.

At the time of this writing, the cost for a Galleri test is $949, and while not covered by most insurance plans, the lab manufacturer, Grail, offers all patients the option of a 12-month payment plan. I am offering this test to anyone who is interested after an initial consultation in our office. Call our office to schedule your consultation: 509-987-1800. If you are not local, the test is available (to US residents, only) through my remote counseling service: *ioeprogram.com/ product/galleri-test-30-minute-lab-review-consult*.

Learn more about the Galleri test at *www.galleri.com*.

## Whole Body MRI

Another tool that can be used for cancer screening is whole body MRI. While not standardly recommended as a cancer screening tool for most individuals, it is very sensitive in being able to identify solid cancers, as well as other conditions such as aneurysms, benign tumors, fatty liver disease, heart disease, and orthopedic issues, throughout the brain and body.

The likelihood of detecting pathological conditions:

- 1–2% of all whole-body MRI scans on asymptomatic individuals detect a cancer (sensitivities and specificities vary)
- 30% of scans detect non-cancer conditions that require additional evaluations

Since the majority of cancer deaths are caused by cancers for which we have no recommended screenings, if you are at high risk of developing cancer (meaning you have a prior and/or family history of cancer, or have tested positive for a genetic mutation that carries cancer), or simply want to do everything you can to detect cancer or other abnormal anatomical concerns, getting a screening whole body MRI is an option for you.

The price range for a whole-body MRI is about $2,000–4,000, and is typically not covered by insurance for most individuals.

# Tracking Your Cancer

Circulating tumor cells (CTCs) are cells that have detached from a primary or metastatic tumor and have begun circulating in the bloodstream. CTCs may travel to other areas and create new tumors in different tissues or organs, a process known as metastasis.

Cancer at any stage can shed tumor cells, as well as fragments of cancer cell DNA (ctDNA or circulating tumor DNA, cfDNA or cell free tumor DNA) or circulating tumor tissue-modified virus (TTMV)-HPV DNA (only with HPV+ cancers) into the blood system. The more advanced the cancer, the more likely tumor cells and their DNA fragments will be found in the blood. Serial CTC, ctDNA/cfDNA, or circulating tumor modified human papilloma virus DNA blood testing ("liquid biopsy") can detect cancer recurrence months to years earlier than radiology scans can. Measuring the presence and number of CTCs or their DNA fragments in the blood can help give prognostic information on treatment efficacy and recurrence risks after treatment.

It's important to note that not all patients with detectable CTCs or their DNA fragments develop a detectable cancer upon subsequent examinations and imaging studies. These cells may be attacked and killed by your body's immune system, they may self-destruct, or they may remain dormant within the body. However, if the conditions are right, they can grow into a detectable tumor. Some of these conditions are:

- suppressed immune system
- systemic inflammation
- insulin resistance
- chronic stress
- excessive free radicals (oxidation)
- stimulation by tumor growth factors/hormones

Researchers are currently studying the clinical use of tailoring cancer treatment, such as chemotherapy and immune therapy, based on the response as measured by following the number of CTCs, ctDNA/cfDNA, or TTMV DNA. This is an exciting area of research, as typically oncologists will give a cancer-killing drug for one to three months before assessing the response to treatment using radiographic scans like PET/CTs, CTs, and MRIs. The use of CTC, ctDNA/cfDNA, or TTMV DNA testing also enables the oncologist to assess response to treatment (such as every one to three months), prompting either a continuation of the current drug regimen or a more rapid change to an alternative drug that might be more effective.

## Signatera ctDNA Test

My preferred ctDNA assay (for tumors that are not HPV+) is the Signatera (Natera) test. Signatera works by having a tiny piece of your original tumor (from a prior or new biopsy) sent to Natera for DNA sequencing to look for mutations that are only found in your tumor. Once these mutations are known (your tumor's DNA fingerprint), a simple blood test can look for the presence and quantity of that ctDNA in your blood over time. A negative result ("ctDNA negative") indicates your cancer is in remission, but a positive result ("ctDNA positive") is a sign of cancer in the body. Signatera has been shown to identify cancer recurrence or progression months before it can be seen on imaging.

Additionally, the test quantifies the amount of ctDNA present, which is helpful in assessing response to treatment. Instead of waiting months for radiology studies to detect progression, a rising ctDNA level can be detected within weeks, prompting your oncologist to make more rapid changes in your treatment. For example, immunotherapy drugs work in fewer than 20% of patients, and it can take months to know whether your treatment is working. Signatera can help you find out if your immunotherapy is working long before changes are seen on imaging.

Signatera can be ordered for any solid cancer for which we have tissue sample from a prior biopsy or surgery. Did you know that the FDA requires pathology laboratories to keep tissue samples from biopsies and surgeries for 10 years? So even if your biopsy or surgery was done years ago, you may still be eligible for Signatera testing.

## How Often Do We Recommend Testing?

I recommend getting a baseline Signatera test (before or during treatment), then retest every two to three months for one to two years, then every six months for up to five years, and then annually. There is no standard ordering frequency for retesting, and will vary, patient to patient, depending on their circumstances. For more information about the Signatera test, visit *www.natera.com/oncology/signatera-advanced-cancer-detection.*

Learn about Signatera billing here: *www.natera.com/oncology/billing.*

## NavDx® Test (for HPV+ Cancers)

NavDx is a groundbreaking blood test that uses proprietary technology to detect and quantify fragments of circulating tumor tissue-modified virus (TTMV) DNA. This unique biomarker has been clinically validated as a powerful tool for the early detection of HPV-driven cancer, making NavDx an essential tool for clinicians across the care continuum.

Whether you are monitoring disease progression or investigating symptoms, NavDx® provides accurate, reliable results that can help guide treatment decisions in real time. Similar to the Signatera test, the NavDX test can:

- Assess treatment response, detecting the presence and quantity of residual disease during and after treatment
- Be used during routine cancer surveillance to detect a recurrence—it detects recurrence a median of four months earlier than would present clinically in a PET or CT scan—to facilitate earlier treatment; 94% positive predictive value, 100% negative predictive value

NavDx® is covered by many insurances. Learn more about the NavDx® test here: *naveris.com/what-is-navdx*.

# Your Risk of Cardiovascular Disease

Did you know that, according to a U.S. population-based study of cancer patients, cardiovascular disease (CVD) is one of the leading causes of death among cancer survivors and that adult cancer survivors had a 42% greater risk of developing cardiovascular disease than people without cancer?[29] The reasons are numerous, including cardiotoxic cancer treatments, physical deconditioning, increased sedentary lifestyle, continued smoking, diabetes, and obesity.

Here, we review the main laboratory testing risk factors in developing cardiovascular disease. You don't want to beat your cancer, only to die of heart disease.

## Lab Tests for CVD Risk Factors

These are the four of the most important CVD risk factor lab tests:
- Total cholesterol
- HDL cholesterol
- ApoB (apolipoprotein-b)

---

[29] Roberta Florido et al., *Cardiovascular Disease Risk Among Cancer Survivors: The Atherosclerosis Risk in Communities (ARIC) Study*, Journal of the American College of Cardiology, Vol. 80, No. 1, pp. 22–32, https://www.jacc.org/doi/10.1016/j.jacc.2022.04.042.

- Lp(a) (lipoprotein-a)

Total cholesterol levels:
- Optimal: <200 mg/dL
- Borderline: 200–240 mg/dL
- Increased risk: >240 mg/dL

HDL cholesterol levels:
- Optimal: >50 mg/dL (male), >60 mg/dL (female)
- Borderline: 40–50 mg/dL (male), 50–60 mg/dL (female)
- Increased risk: <40 mg/dL (male), <50 mg/dL (female)

ApoB
- Optimal: <80 mg/dL
- Borderline: 80–120 mg/dL
- Increased risk: >120 mg/dL

In a 2019 review article in *JAMA Cardiology*,[30] Allan Sniderman and his colleagues make the case that apolipoprotein B (apoB) level—rather than LDL, non-HDL-cholesterol, or even LDL particle count (LDL-P)—is the best measure of potentially atherogenic lipoproteins. A greater number of apoB-containing particles leads to a greater number of these particles that enter and get trapped within the wall of the artery, leading to a greater amount of injury to the arterial wall. One such test for your apolipoprotein B (apoB) level is one from Boston Heart Diagnostics (see *bostonheartdiagnostics.com/test/apolipoprotein-b-apob*).

Lp(a)
- Optimal: <30 mg/dL
- Borderline: 30–50 mg/dL
- Increased: risk >50 mg/dL

---

30 Allan D. Sniderman, et al., "Apolipoprotein B Particles and Cardiovascular Disease: A Narrative Review," *JAMA Cardiology*, 2019, Vol. 4, Issue 12, pp. 1287–95, jamanetwork.com/journals/jamacardiology/article-abstract/2753612.

The Lp(a) test only needs to be performed once, since its level does not change much over one's lifetime. It's estimated that about one in five people in the U.S. has an Lp(a) level that puts them at risk for heart disease. Having an elevated Lp(a) is genetically inherited. One example of this test is also by Boston Heart Diagnostics (*bostonheartdiagnostics.com/test/ lipoproteina-lpa*).

Other important CVD risk factor lab tests are:
Fibrinogen:
- Optimal: <370 mg/dL
- Borderline: 370–470 mg/dL
- Increased risk: >470 mg/dL

High-sensitivity C-reactive protein (hsCRP):
- Optimal: <1 mg/L
- Borderline: 1–3 mg/L
- Increased risk: >3 mg/L

Homocysteine:
- Optimal: <10 umol/L
- Borderline: 10–14 umol/L
- Increased risk: >14 umol/L

Oral glucose tolerance test (OGTT) with insulin
- Fasting glucose: <90 mg/dL
- Fasting insulin: <6 mIU/L
- Oral glucose tolerance test (OGTT) 1-hour glucose: <130 mg/dL
- OGTT with insulin: 1-hour insulin: <30 mIU/L
- OGTT 2-hour glucose: <100 mg/dL
- OGTT with insulin: 2-hour insulin: <20 mIU/L

HbA1c
- Optimal: </=5.1%

## Other Important CVD Risk Factors

Other important factors that indicate you may be at risk for cardiovascular disease are:

- High blood pressure—Track over time
- Insulin resistance and type 2 diabetes—Track over time
- Cigarette smoking—Quit!
- Limit alcohol consumption
- Being overweight or obese—Track over time
- Not being physically active—Focus on both muscle mass building and aerobic fitness
- Family history of early heart disease, heart attacks, or stroke

To estimate your risk of developing CVD, there are two helpful CVD risk calculators, one which can be found at *www.cvriskcalculator.com*, and the other at *www.mesa-nhlbi.org/MESACHDRisk/MesaRiskScore/RiskScore.aspx*. To use these, you will need to know your:

- Total cholesterol
- HDL cholesterol
- Systolic blood pressure
- Coronary artery calcification score (optional)
- Gender, age, race, history of diabetes, smoking status, family history of heart attack, and if you're taking any lipid- and/or blood pressure-lowering medications

I recommend that you share your risk assessment score with your primary care provider, as this can help them in their counseling and management of this risk.

## What Is a CAC Test?

You may want to get a coronary artery calcification (CAC) test to find out your CAC score, a measure of the amount of calcification in your coronary arteries. This radiology study is a special type of CT scan of your heart. CAC testing may also be called:

- Calcium Scan of the Heart
- Coronary Calcium Score
- Cardiac Scoring
- Cardiac CT for Calcium Scoring
- Calcium Scan Test

The test result is given as a number, called a CAC score. It can range from 0 to over 400. The more evidence of calcium and thickening that is seen in the inside lining of the arteries, the higher the score. The higher your CAC score, the more likely you are to develop heart disease, or have an event such as a heart attack or stroke.

A coronary calcium scan is often done in a hospital or other medical imaging facility. The test:

- Is fairly quick (it takes about 10–20 minutes to complete)
- Uses a low dose radiation CT scan
- Doesn't require contrast (a special dye injected in your vein as in other imaging tests)
- Often includes an electrocardiogram (ECG)

CAC testing is not recommended if you are already known to have a high risk for coronary heart disease (CHD), have heart disease already, or if you've had a heart attack, stroke, or stent or bypass surgery. Learn more about this test here, or visit *www.cardiosmart.org/Heart-Conditions/High-Cholesterol/Content/Coronary-Artery-Calcium-Scoring*.

Use this simple calculator (*www.mesa-nhlbi.org/Calcium/input.aspx*) to find out how your CAC score compares with others your age.

I recommend that anyone—not just those with a history of cancer—who is interested in assessing their risk of a future cardiovascular event consider getting a coronary artery calcium CT scan, in addition to assessing other risk factors.

I follow these Mayo Clinic recommendations.

### Who should get a calcium-score screening?

You should consider a calcium scan if you are between the ages of 40 and 70 and at increased risk for heart disease but do not have symptoms. People at increased risk include those with the following traits:

- Family history of heart disease
- Past or present smoker
- History of high cholesterol, diabetes, or high blood pressure
- Overweight
- Inactive lifestyle
- Any abnormal CVD risk factor lab test results (see above)

If you are less than 40 years old and high cholesterol runs in your family (familial hypercholesterolemia), you might consider a calcium scan.

**Note:** Because there are certain forms of coronary disease—such as "soft plaque" atherosclerosis—that escape detection during this CT scan, it is important to remember that this test is not absolute in predicting your risk for a life-threatening event, such as a heart attack.

## High Blood Pressure Increases Your Risk for CVD

Measuring your blood pressure has to be done correctly or it won't be accurate. Learn more about this at *www.heart.org/en/health-topics/high-blood-pressure/understanding-blood-pressure-readings/monitoring-your-blood-pressure-at-home*.

Ranges and Management:

- Normal: <120 mm Hg (systolic) and <80 mm Hg (diastolic)
- Elevated: 120–129 mm Hg (systolic) and <80 mm Hg (diastolic); lifestyle changes recommended
- Stage 1 Hypertension: 130–139 mm Hg (systolic) or 80–89 mm Hg (diastolic); lifestyle changes recommended +/- blood pressure medications
- Stage 2 Hypertension: >/=140 mm Hg (systolic) or >/=90 mm Hg (diastolic); lifestyle changes recommended + blood pressure medications
- Stage 3 Hypertension: >180 mm Hg (systolic) and/or >120 mm Hg (diastolic)—*call your health care provider immediately!* Lifestyle changes recommended + blood pressure medications

What should you do if you have any of these CVD risk factors?

- Talk with your primary care provider (PCP) about management recommendations
- Ask your PCP to refer you to a cardiologist if your 10-year risk of CVD is 5% or higher (see links to online calculators on page 104)
- Ask your PCP to refer you to see a cardiologist if your Lp(a) or apoB are in the increased risk group (see p. 102)
- If you are overweight or have insulin resistance, refer back to the section on insulin resistance, starting on page 21
- Focus on optimizing your overall health:
  - Get better sleep
  - Reduce stress
  - Exercise
  - Improve your gut health
  - Minimize toxins

- Use functional medicine testing to assess your underlying physiological status and make targeted changes to improve any deficiencies and abnormalities

# Cardio-Oncology

Cardio-oncology is a relatively new field of medicine that is concerned with the detection, monitoring, and treatment of cardiovascular disease that may occur as a side effect of cancer treatment. Both chemotherapy and radiotherapy can cause cardiac dysfunction, which is a major cause of morbidity and mortality in cancer patients.

Certain cancer drugs have cardiotoxic side effects that are well known to your oncologist, which is why they may test your heart prior to, during, and after treatment with these drugs. These tests can include echocardiograms and MUGA scans to assess heart rate and rhythm and the health of your heart muscle and heart valves. Depending on the drugs your oncologist plans to use, they will first discuss their risks and how they will monitor you and screen for cardiac side effects.

Despite advances in the targeting and effectiveness of radiation therapy, side effects can develop over the years due to the late effects of radiation on blood vessels in the treated body locations.

*Have you had radiation treatment to the brain or head and neck?* If so, your risk of having a future stroke may be as high as 40%. Possible conditions include cerebrovascular and carotid disease, thyroid dysfunction, and autonomic (nervous system) dysfunction, which are diagnosed by physical exam and various tests, such as imaging (CT, MRI, CTA, and MRA), carotid ultrasound, and a thyroid TSH blood test. If your neck was previously radiated, a carotid ultrasound may be recommended (one year after treatment and every five years after that).

*Have you had radiation treatment to the lung or chest?* If so, your risk of developing or worsening heart disease may be higher than expected. Possible conditions include atherosclerosis of any blood vessel, valvular and/or pericardial disease, and heart failure. In addition to a physical exam to determine bilateral blood pressure, any signs of SVC (superior vena cava) syndrome, checking the jugular venous pressure, and detecting any abnormal heart sounds (murmurs, rubs, and/or gallops), diagnostic tests may be prescribed, including imaging (CT, MRI, CAC, and CTA), EKG/ECG, and stress testing. If your chest was radiated, a heart ultrasound may be recommended (6–12 months after treatment and every five years after that).

*Have you undergone radiation treatment to the pelvic/ abdominal region?* If so, your risk of peripheral artery disease may be increased. Conditions include aorto-iliac atherosclerosis and renovascular hypertension. Physical exams including an ankle brachial index and blood pressure monitoring may be performed, and tests, such as a renal ultrasound and serum creatinine blood test, may be recommended.

These are just some of the long-term risks associated with radiation treatment, which, in addition to routine scheduled cancer surveillance (such as radiology studies, lab tests and physical exams), is why it's important to continue to follow up with your radiation oncologist to be evaluated for your potential risks. If cardiovascular abnormalities are identified on screening, a referral to cardiology (or cardio-oncology subspecialist) is the next step.

# Cancer Survivorship Care Plan

The good news for cancer survivorship is that the numbers are growing, with an estimated 17 million survivors living in the United States alone. Unfortunately, cancer treatments are not without consequence, and these survivors may live with the long-term effects of treatments. The Institute of Medicine (IOM) researched the state of care for cancer survivors and found that little guidance is available for survivors and their healthcare providers to overcome the medical and psychosocial problems that may arise after treatment.

The IOM suggests that once a person has completed cancer therapy, they should be provided with a summary of the treatments received and a follow-up care plan. *This care plan should summarize the potential late effects, their prevention, symptoms, and treatment, cancer screening recommendations, psychosocial effects, financial issues, recommendations for a healthy lifestyle, genetic counseling, referrals for follow-up care, and a list of support resources.* While this plan is extremely important, the resources required to create it have made it hard to incorporate into practice.

# What information do I need to create a cancer survivorship care plan?

The OncoLife™ Survivorship Care Plan[31] is a survivorship care plan that is tailored to you, based on the answers you provide in a brief questionnaire. In order to develop the most accurate plan of care, you may need to talk to your oncology team to have some details of your cancer therapy available. Information includes:

- Type of cancer
- If you underwent surgery, what procedures were done
- If you received chemotherapy, what medications were received
- If you received radiation therapy, what type of cancer was this done for

# How do I use my survivorship care plan?

This care plan is for you to review and discuss with your healthcare team (both oncology and primary care). Keep in mind that every case is different and the risks of some side effects vary, based on the actual dose of radiation or chemotherapy you received, and/or the techniques used to administer these therapies to you. It is very important to review your care plan with your oncology team to further clarify your risk.

---

31   See https://oncolife.oncolink.org/form/oncolife_v11.

# What if I survived a childhood cancer?

The OncoLife™ Survivorship Care Plan program (*smartalacc. oncolink.org*) is designed for survivors of adult cancers.

Childhood cancer survivors have been studied in greater detail and much more is known about the late effects of treatment during childhood development. The Children's Oncology Group website, *childrensoncologygroup.org*, is a wonderful resource for survivors of childhood cancers. In addition, childhood cancer survivors should encourage their healthcare team to review the extensive guidelines for long-term care (*childrensoncologygroup.org/index. php/survivorshipguidelines*) developed by the Children's Oncology Group.

# How I Apply Functional and Precision Medicine Testing: A Sample Case

My patient is a 60-year-old female who has been diagnosed with a left-sided breast cancer (invasive ductal carcinoma, grade 3, estrogen and progesterone receptors positive, HER-2 negative). The tumor measures 5.5 centimeters in maximal dimension on breast MRI. She has multiple irregular-appearing left axillary lymph nodes noted on MRI, and one has been biopsied and confirmed to be involved with metastatic breast carcinoma. Her cancer's stage is a clinical IIIA (cT3N1aM0).

Based on the large size of her tumor, the oncology team has recommended treating her with a course of chemotherapy, upfront ("neoadjuvant"), to make the tumor more easily resectable by shrinking it. This also allows the oncology team to assess the response of the tumor to the chemotherapy drugs. (If the tumor shrinks during chemotherapy, we continue this regimen; if the tumor gets larger, we would switch to another regimen.) She completes a course of neoadjuvant chemotherapy, with a weekly regimen of carboplatin and paclitaxel, with immunotherapy (pembrolizumab, given every three weeks), followed by more chemotherapy: dose-dense doxorubicin and cyclophosphamide.

After completion of her neoadjuvant regimen, she undergoes another breast MRI, which shows a partial response to treatment. The tumor now measures 4 cm in size, and while the left axillary lymph nodes are still present, they are now slightly less prominent.

She undergoes a left-sided mastectomy and axillary lymph node dissection and prophylactic right-sided mastectomy. The pathology notes: 1) a 4.5-cm residual invasive ductal carcinoma tumor in the left breast; 2) one out of 18 left axillary lymph nodes were involved with carcinoma; and 3) a 2-mm extranodal extension (meaning metastatic cancer has invaded through the capsule of the lymph node and into the surrounding fat). Her pathological stage is a IIA (ypT2N1aM0). Her right breast pathology is benign. She then continues on immunotherapy, to complete a one-year course of pembrolizumab.

It is at this point that the patient, herself, decides to see me for an integrative oncology consultation. We discuss numerous topics during her consultation:

- Personal medical history (high blood pressure, left-sided breast cancer)
- Family medical history (numerous relatives with cardiovascular disease and type 2 diabetes; no family history of breast, ovarian, colorectal, prostate, pancreatic, or other cancers)
- Social history (retired school teacher; lifelong nonsmoker; 2–4 glasses of wine a week)
- She indicates that she always tries to eat a healthful, omnivorous diet (vegetables, meat, fish, poultry, eggs) and exercises when she has the time; she has gained about 20 pounds since entering menopause (at age 52)
- She sleeps about six hours per night
- No medication allergies
- She states that since completing her chemotherapy and mastectomies, she has been very tired; she has also

noticed that her left arm recently feels a bit heavier in comparison to her right arm, and she has decreased range of motion in her left shoulder due to tightness

- On exam, I note that she has well-healed mastectomy scars and mild fullness in the appearance of her left upper and lower arm; her right arm has decreased range of motion when raised, due to tightness in the muscles and joint of her left chest and shoulder; the rest of her examination is normal

Her goal for today's visit is to learn more about ways to optimize her overall health and hopefully reduce her risk for cancer recurrence. After taking her medical history and doing a physical examination, I discuss multiple topics with her regarding nutrition, exercise, stress management, sleep, and functional medicine testing.

To address the possibility of lymphedema (swelling in the tissues due to her lymph node surgery) in her left arm, and to evaluate the decreased range of motion in her left arm/shoulder, I place a referral for her to see a physical therapist who is a certified lymphedema therapist, someone who specializes in lymphedema therapy.

She is also interested in using the Signatera test to help in the early detection of a cancer recurrence. I order a baseline Signatera, which we will recheck over time. Additionally, even though she has no known family history of cancer, I recommend that she get a hereditary cancer genetic test. When ordering the hereditary cancer genetic test, I recommend a multi-gene panel assay that looks for abnormalities in many different genes to cast a wider net to assess for one's genetic cancer risks for various cancers. Any identified abnormalities should be reviewed with the patient by a genetic counselor.

We then decide to assess her nutrient status (NutrEval test), HPA axis function, and estrogen metabolites (DUTCH test), gut health (GI MAP assay), insulin sensitivity (A1c, insulin-glucose response test), and systemic inflammatory status (hsCRP, IL-6 and fibrinogen).

## Test Results

**Signatera: POSITIVE (20.56 MTM/mL)**

While she has no detectable evidence of cancer based on her physical examination, this indicates the presence of cancer cells somewhere in her body.

I contact her medical oncologist and let them know about this result and my plan to recheck the Signatera test in six weeks. If this shows an increase in the quantity of circulating tumor DNA, I will order either a PET/CT or a CT of the chest, abdomen, and pelvis (CT CAP), to look for evidence that cancer has recurred.

Unfortunately, six weeks later, her Signatera again comes back POSITIVE, and this time it's higher (29.10 MTM/mL). Her physical exam is again normal and she has no new symptoms.

Her insurance won't cover the PET-CT, so I order a CT CAP instead. The CT shows numerous, new sub-centimeter lung nodules, bilaterally. A CT-guided needle biopsy of one of these nodules confirms metastatic breast carcinoma. This prompts her medical oncologist to start her on a new drug regimen for metastatic breast cancer.

**Color hereditary cancer genetic mutation panel:** Negative for mutations

**GI MAP assay:**
- No dysbiosis
- Digestive enzymes: Normal
- Secretory IgA: Low – Low levels of these IgA antibodies can lead to an impaired gut immune response to infectious organisms; one main cause for low IgA is chronic stress

- Calprotectin: High – This is a biomarker for gut inflammation and can be caused by dysbiosis (although not in her case), food sensitivities, chronic stress, toxins, medications, and many other factors
- Zonulin: High – This is a biomarker for "leaky gut," a condition in which the tight junctions between intestinal lining cells have become permeable, i.e., organisms, proteins, and toxins are now more easily able to cross into the blood; leaky gut increases nutrient leakage from the blood into the stool. These conditions can lead to systemic inflammation, immune system exhaustion, increased toxic burden on the body, and nutrient deficiencies.

I recommend food sensitivity testing or doing a restriction–reintroduction diet to identify potential foods that may be causing sensitivity reactions, gut inflammation, and leaky gut. I also recommend starting her on a three-month course of a gut-healing supplement to address gut inflammation and leaky gut. She opts to do a restriction–reintroduction diet.

I also recommend retesting with another GI MAP assay in 6–12 months to see if things have improved with her interventions.

**DUTCH test:**
- Cortisol: Low (total daily cortisol and daytime cortisol levels) – This is a sign of HPA axis dysfunction, where the normal daily production of cortisol can diminish over time, the most common cause being chronic stress; other possible causes include poor sleep, nutrient deficiencies, too little or too much exercise, gut dysbiosis, and many others
- Methylation activity: Normal
- Estrogen metabolites: Normal (Had her 2-OH estrogen metabolite been below the normal range, I would have recommended a diet rich in cruciferous vegetables, or

a sulforaphane supplement, to increase this estrogen receptor "protective" metabolite)

- Melatonin: Normal

I counsel her on stress management and how she can improve her sleep from 6 hours per night to 6.5 to optimally 8 hours per night. (Sleep hygiene is discussed in the more comprehensive book *Empowered Against Cancer*.)

**NutrEval test:**
- Antioxidants: Low for vitamins A, C, E, alpha lipoic acid, glutathione, and plant-based antioxidants
- B vitamins: Low for B1, B3, B6, B9, B12
- Minerals: Low for magnesium
- Omega-3 fatty acids: Low
- Vitamin D: 71 – Normal

I counsel her on nutrient repletion through diet (preferred) and/or supplements. I offer a referral to a dietitian and discuss with her the Optimising Nutrition Macronutrient and Micronutrient online programs (see page 38).

**Insulin sensitivity testing:**
- A1c: 5.2% – while within the accepted range, our target goal is 5.1% or lower
- Fasting glucose: 88 – Normal
- Stimulated glucose: 139 – Normal
- Fasting insulin: 28.4 – High
- Stimulated insulin: 463 – High

I explain that while her A1c and fasting glucose levels look quite good, the insulin levels are too high, which implies that she has insulin resistance. I counsel her on the risks of insulin resistance and how to address it, and tell her that the dietitian will discuss this with her as well. I also recommend the Optimising Nutrition Data Driven Fasting online program to help coach her on how to reverse her insulin resistance (see page 27).

**Systemic inflammation:**
- hsCRP: High (2.5)
- IL-6: Normal
- Fibrinogen: High

I counsel her on the risks and potential causes of systemic inflammation: nutrient deficiencies, insulin resistance, getting not enough or too much exercise, poor sleep, dysbiosis, toxic burden, and chronic stress. Addressing these will hopefully reduce her systemic inflammation.

In my opinion, running tests such as these and addressing any abnormalities does not directly improve cancer outcomes. What it does do, however, is help our patients optimize numerous health variables that contribute to their metabolic health, immune health, and others that indirectly influence cancer outcomes, chronic diseases, and quality of life.

# My Final Thoughts for You

As a practicing radiation oncologist, integrative oncologist, and functional medicine provider, I see patients every day in the clinic who are undergoing conventional oncological therapies. They are also receiving integrative care to address not only the side effects and symptoms of their cancer treatment but also try to improve overall health outcomes and, possibly, cancer outcomes.

While we do not yet have robust studies to prove that this comprehensive approach is superior to simply applying a conventional-only oncological therapeutic approach, it is well established that when we have insulin resistance, systemic inflammation, gut microbiome dysbiosis, sleep problems, chronic stress, and excessive toxic load, that these conditions may indirectly impact our cancer outcomes, general health, and quality of life. Therefore, why not try to optimize these underlying conditions when detected before, during, and after cancer treatment? My hope is that more research will be done to validate the use of functional medicine testing, self-tracking (sleep, diet, HRV, etc.), and precision medicine testing as important components to overall cancer care and survivorship.

The information in this guidebook merely scratches the surface on how we can use these state-of-the-art tools to help personalize and guide interventions to improve health outcomes. If you want to incorporate these into your cancer care, I recommend seeking a functional medicine trained practitioner with experience working with cancer patients to be part of your team.

# Resources

Dr. Brian Lawenda offers in-person and remote integrative oncology consultations to patients worldwide. To learn more and schedule a consultation, visit *ioeprogram.com/consultations*.

*Empowered Against Cancer* by Brian Lawenda, MD and Conner Middelmann, the foundational cancer treatment book that this book builds upon: *www.amazon.com/Empowered-Against-Cancer-Science-Based-Strategies-ebook/dp/B09T28X6BQ*. See also this book's site, *FMFCancer.com*, for more information and for printable copies of the forms that appear at the end of this book.

Dr. Lawenda's three recipe books for meal ideas to help cancer patients and survivors, one for those who need to gain weight, one for those looking to lose weight, and one for those who wish to maintain their current healthy weight: *optimisingnutrition.com/optimal-nutrition-for-cancer-management*.

Conner Middelmann's Modern Mediterranean Diet website: *modernmediterranean.com*.

## Apps and Devices

Cronometer calorie tracking: *cronometer.com*

Meditation, to reduce mental stress and improve well-being:

- 10 Percent Happier: *www.tenpercent.com*
- Calm: *www.calm.com*
- Headspace: *www.headspace.com/meditation/sleep*

Biofeedback tool using heart rate variability (HRV) to track stress levels: *store.heartmath.com/inner-balance*

EWG Healthy Living app (*www.ewg.org/apps*) provides suggestions on the least toxic food items and personal and baby products

## Calculators and Assessment Tools

Cancer risk calculators for common cancers: *www.calculators.org/health/cancer.php*

Calorie assessment tool Body Weight Planner from the National Institute of Health's National Institutes of Diabetes and Digestive and Kidney Diseases: *www.niddk.nih.gov/bwp*

"Reduce My Risk"—How to reduce your risk of many types of cancer: *risk.oncolink.org*

Ideal body weight calculator:
*www.calculator.net/ideal-weight-calculator.html*
(Males should use the Devine formula and females use the Robinson formula.)

Convert pounds to kilograms:
*www.calculator.net/weight-calculator.html*
(or simply divide your weight in pounds by 2.2 to get your weight in kilograms)

Estimate your body fat percentage using age, sex, height, neck circumference, and waist circumference: *www.calculator.net/body-fat-calculator.html*

Calculating BMI, body mass index (body fat): *www.calculator.net/bmi-calculator.html* using age, gender, height, and weight (While BMI is not the best assessment tool to determine how overweight, underweight, or of normal weight you are, increased BMI has been linked to many chronic health conditions, e.g., type 2 diabetes, cardiovascular disease, and cancer.)

WHtR/waist–height ratio:
*www.omnicalculator.com/health/waist-height-ratio*— this measures your body fat distribution, which correlates more closely than BMI with most health outcomes

Assess your acute (short-term) stress using the National Comprehensive Cancer Network's risk assessment questionnaire, NCCN Distress

Thermometer: *www.nccn.org/docs/default-source/ patient-resources/nccn_distress_thermometer.pdf*

CVD risk assessment calculator: *www.cvriskcalculator.com*

CVD Risk Assessment MESA risk score: *www.mesa-nhlbi.org/MESACHDRisk/ MesaRiskScore/RiskScore.aspx*

CAC (coronary artery calcium) testing: *www.cardiosmart.org/Heart-Conditions/High- Cholesterol/Content/Coronary-Artery-Calcium- Scoring*

Find out how your CAC score compares with others your age: *www.mesa-nhlbi.org/Calcium/input.aspx*

## Food/Diet Guidance

*Empowered Against Cancer*: *www.amazon.com/ Empowered-Against-Cancer-Science-Based- Strategies-ebook/dp/B09T28X6BQ*

Three nutrient-dense recipe books for cancer patients: *optimisingnutrition.com/nutrient-dense- foods-meals-cancer/#h-the-recipe-books* for gaining weight, losing weight, or maintaining your optimal weight

Conner Middelmann's Modern Mediterranean Diet website: *modernmediterranean.com*

Low-FODMAP Diet:

- *integrativeoncology-essentials.com/2019/10/ low-fodmap-diet-reduces-gi-inflammation*
- Monash University's FODMAP Diet Guide: *www.monashfodmap.com* (see also its app feature under Apps)

Improve your diet, particularly through micronutrient and macronutrient intakes: *optimisingnutrition.com/micros-masterclass* and *optimisingnutrition.com/macros-masterclass*

Environmental Working Group's annual list of cleanest and dirtiest fruits and vegetables (best and worst for pesticide contamination): *www.ewg.org/foodnews*

EWG Consumer Guide on how to choose less toxic seafood: *www.ewg.org/research/ewgs-good-seafood-guide*

Monterey Bay Aquarium Seafood Watch Guides: *www.seafoodwatch.org/seafood-recommendations/ consumer-guides* to help select the most environmentally sustainable options

## Lab Tests

Galleri multi-cancer early detection test: *www. galleri.com/the-galleri-test/types-of-cancer-detected*. (Dr. Lawenda offers this test in person and also to U.S. residents via his remote counseling service; see *ioeprogram.com/product/galleri-test-30-minute-lab-review-consult*)

Advanced cancer detection: Signatera ctDNA Test, *www.natera.com/oncology/signatera-advanced-cancer-detection*

DNA cancer test to detect HPV-driven cancers: NavDx® test: *naveris.com/what-is-navdx*

To assess toxic load:

- Genova NutrEval (in addition to nutrient testing, this reports toxic metals): *ioeprogram.com/product/micronutrient-test-vitamin-d-genova-diagnostics-nutreval*

- Mosaic Diagnostics GPL-TOX: *ioeprogram.com/product/toxic-non-metal-chemical-exposure-urine*

- Mosaic Diagnostics MycoTOX: *ioeprogram.com/product/mycotox-profile-mold-exposure-urine*

- Quicksilver Scientific: Mercury tri-test & blood metals panel for heavy metals testing

To assess methylation activity and estrogen metabolites:

- DUTCH Test: *ioeprogram.com/product/dutch-plus*

To assess drug sensitivity:

- EVA-PCD Functional Profile (aka Ex-Vivo Analysis of Programmed Cell Death), see *www.nagourneycancerinstitute.com* or call 800-542-4357

- Paris test: *senginemedicine.com/paris-test*

- ASC Oncology test: *www.asc-oncology.com/en/home*

Food intolerances:

- Dr. Lawenda's Food Sensitivity Questionnaire (see page 136)

- Dr. Lawenda's Symptom Tracker Worksheet (see page 137)

- Cyrex 10 Multiple Food Immune Reactivity Screen (*ioeprogram.com/lab-tests*), a high-quality IgG and IgA food intolerance test which also assesses immune reactions to foods, raw and/or modified, food enzymes, lectins, and artificial food additives, colorings, and gums

Apolipoprotein B (apoB) level:
*bostonheartdiagnostics.com/test/apolipoprotein-b-apob*

Lipoprotein(a) or Lp(a) level:
*bostonheartdiagnostics.com/test/lipoproteina-lpa*

## Medication Interactions

To check for potential interactions between medications you're taking: *naturalmedicines.therapeuticresearch.com*

## Online Courses, Videos and Programs

4–7–8 breathing demonstration video: *www.drweil.com/videos-features/videos/breathing-exercises-4-7-8-breath* to immediately reduce stress with a pranayama yoga technique. (See also page 51 for a description of how to perform this.)

Data Driven Fasting course: *www.datadrivenfasting.com* teaches you how to use blood sugar testing to reverse insulin resistance

To improve your diet, notably micronutrient and macronutrient intakes: *optimisingnutrition.com/micros-masterclass* and *optimisingnutrition.com/macros-masterclass*

## Probiotics

FLORÉ Precision Probiotics, Sun Genomics: (*flore.com*)

Fullscript Online Supplement Formulary: 10% discount off all supplements ordered through Dr. Lawenda's affiliate link, *us.fullscript.com/welcome/blawenda* (Affiliate proceeds support the website and administrative management expenses for Dr. Lawenda's educational platforms *ioeprogram.com* and *IntegrativeOncology-Essentials.com*)

## Water and Product Safety Guidance

Campaign for Safe Cosmetics' list of toxic chemicals to avoid, and those found particularly in beauty and personal care products: *www.safecosmetics.org*

Environmental Working Group (EWG) recommendations for the least toxic personal care products, including makeup, sunscreen, and baby products: *www.ewg.org/skindeep*

EWG Guide to Healthy Cleaning to select the least toxic household cleaning products: *www.ewg.org/guides/ cleaners*

EWG's Tap Water Database to evaluate the quality of your drinking water: *www.ewg.org/tapwater*

EWGs Water Filter Guide on how to choose the right filter for your water quality needs and budget: *www.ewg.org/tapwater/water-filter-guide.php*

## Websites, General Information

Detailed reports on the most common cancer diagnoses by Ralph W. Moss, PhD, plus informational and personalized consultations for cancer patients and their families. His 50-page report *The Ultimate Guide to Cancer: DIY Research* is designed to help you research your particular cancer, and is available free of charge at: *www.mossreports.com*

List of integrative oncologists in the US, by state, and Canada, by province: *glennsabin.com/integrative-oncology-providers*

Licensed naturopathic doctors in North America who specialize in oncology: *oncanp.org*

National Cancer Institute (NCI) designated cancer center: *www.cancer.gov/research/nci-role/cancer-centers* (You can also call the NCI Cancer Information Service (1-800-4-CANCER) or consult online with an information specialist through its LiveHelp feature, *livehelp.cancer.gov/app/chat/chat_launch*)

Treatment of Cancer by Type Guidelines, by the National Comprehensive Cancer Network: *www.nccn.org/patientresources/patient-resources/guidelines-for-patients*

National Cancer Institute PDQ (Physician Data Query), *www.cancer.gov/publications/pdq*

Telehealth mental health counseling services:
* Ginger: *www.ginger.com*
* Talkspace: *www.talkspace.com*

CareOncology: cancer prevention programs, early cancer detection, and adjunctive therapies for later-stage cancers: *careoncology.com*

How to measure your blood pressure correctly: *www.heart.org/en/health-topics/high-blood-pressure/understanding-blood-pressure-readings/monitoring-your-blood-pressure-at-home*

Risks and care recommendations following cancer treatment: The OncoLife Survivorship Care Plan (based on your answers to a brief questionnaire), *oncolife.oncolink.org/form/oncolife_v11*

Care plan and recommendations for survivors of adulthood cancers: The OncoLife Survivorship Care Plan: *smartalacc.oncolink.org*

Care recommendations and support for childhood cancer survivors by Children's Oncology Group: *childrensoncologygroup.org* (Be sure to review the extensive guidelines for long-term care, *childrensoncologygroup.org/index.php/survivorshipguidelines*)

How to Starve Cancer: book and course by Jane McLelland, *www.howtostarvecancer.com*

# Food Sensitivity Questionnaire

| Category | Symptom | Score |
|---|---|---|
| ENERGY | Fatigue, sluggishness | |
| | Apathy, lethargy | |
| | Hyperactivity | |
| | Restlessness | |
| | TOTAL | |
| DIGESTION | Nausea | |
| | Constant fullness | |
| | Diarrhea | |
| | Constipation | |
| | Bloated feeling | |
| | Belching, burping | |
| | Passing gas, flatulence | |
| | Heartburn | |
| | Intestinal or stomach pain. Which? | |
| | TOTAL | |
| MIND | Poor memory | |
| | Confusion | |
| | Poor concentration or focus | |
| | difficulty making decisions | |
| | TOTAL | |

| Category | Symptom | Score |
|---|---|---|
| SKIN | Acne | |
| | Hives or other allergic breakout | |
| | Rash or persistently dry skin | |
| | Hair loss | |
| | Flushing or hot flashes | |
| | Frequently feel cold | |
| | Excessive sweating | |
| | Part of body frequently feels numb | |
| | TOTAL | |
| NOSE | Stuffy nose | |
| | Sinus problems | |
| | Hay fever | |
| | Sneezing attacks | |
| | Excessive mucus | |
| | TOTAL | |

SCORING  <2 food sensitivity unlikely
2–4 possible food sensitivity
4–6 likely food sensitivity
>6 probably food sensitivity

No matter where you scored, an elimination diet can help you determine the most common foods that could be causing your symptoms. I recommend you remove those foods for at least 3 weeks, and then reintroduce them one at a time to see which foods may be causing a reaction.

## Food Restriction & Reintroduction Symptom Tracker

| Symptom(s) | Day 1 | Day 2 | Day 3 |
|---|---|---|---|
| Digestive/Bowel Function | | | |
| Bladder/ Kidney Function | | | |
| Joint/Muscle Aches | | | |
| Congestion/Runny Nose | | | |
| Headache/Sinus Pressure | | | |
| Skin Reactions, Flushing, Sweating, Feeling Cold | | | |
| Energy Level/Fatigue | | | |
| Sleep Quality & Length | | | |
| Mental Alertness/Brain Fog | | | |
| Additional Symptoms | | | |

www.ingramcontent.com/pod-product-compliance
Lightning Source LLC
Chambersburg PA
CBHW041041050426
42335CB00056B/3243